ANX

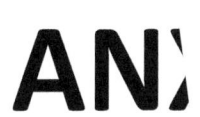

Self Help Guide to Reduce Depression, Overcome Jealousy, Couple Conflicts and Kick Negative Thinking

(Eliminate Fear of Abandonment and Improve Communication)

Jenny Duff

Published by Kevin Dennis

© **Jenny Duff**

All Rights Reserved

Anxiety in Relationship: Self Help Guide to Reduce Depression, Overcome Jealousy, Couple Conflicts and Kick Negative Thinking (Eliminate Fear of Abandonment and Improve Communication)

ISBN 978-1-989920-65-7

All rights reserved. No part of this guide may be reproduced in any form without permission in writing from the publisher except in the case of brief quotations embodied in critical articles or reviews.

Legal & Disclaimer

The information contained in this book is not designed to replace or take the place of any form of medicine or professional medical advice. The information in this book has been provided for educational and entertainment purposes only.

The information contained in this book has been compiled from sources deemed reliable, and it is accurate to the best of the Author's knowledge; however, the Author cannot guarantee its accuracy and validity and cannot be held liable for any errors or omissions. Changes are periodically made to this book. You must consult your doctor or get professional medical advice before using any of the suggested remedies, techniques, or information in this book.

Upon using the information contained in this book, you agree to hold harmless the Author from and against any damages, costs, and expenses, including any legal fees potentially resulting from the application of any of the information provided by this guide. This disclaimer applies to any damages or injury caused by the use and application, whether directly or indirectly, of any advice or information presented, whether for breach of contract, tort, negligence, personal injury, criminal intent, or under any other cause of action.

You agree to accept all risks of using the information presented inside this book. You need to consult a professional medical practitioner in order to ensure you are both able and healthy enough to participate in this program.

Table of Contents

INTRODUCTION 1

CHAPTER 1: EVALUATE WHAT YOU LOSE WHEN YOU FAIL TO DEFY YOUR SHYNESS 2

CHAPTER 2: INTERMEDIATE TECHNIQUES 5

CHAPTER 3: STEP 1: DETERMINE WHETHER YOU HAVE AN ANXIETY DISORDER 10

CHAPTER 4: SOCIAL ANXIETY 16

CHAPTER 5: WHY SHOULD YOU SPEND YOUR TIME TO READ ALL THESE PAGES? 24

CHAPTER 6: DEPRESSION AND ITS COMPLICATIONS 29

CHAPTER 7: ACCEPTANCE 34

CHAPTER 8: USING A MANTRA 39

CHAPTER 9: THERAPIES 44

CHAPTER 10: SO, WHAT'S THE SECRET INGREDIENT? 47

CHAPTER 11: HOW TO COMBAT ANXIETY AND AVOID PANIC ATTACKS 50

CHAPTER 12: OTHER ALTERNATIVE THERAPIES FOR ANXIETY 66

CHAPTER 13: HOW ANXIETY AFFIRMATIONS CAN ALLEVIATE DISORDERS 70

CHAPTER 14: RELAXATION TECHNIQUES 76

- CHAPTER 15: LET'S GET STARTED 81
- CHAPTER 16: FUN ACTIVITIES 88
- CHAPTER 17: TRICKS OF THE MIND.................. 92
- CHAPTER 18: SUPPLEMENTS FOR DEPRESSION AND ANXIETY 96
- CHAPTER 19: SECTION TWO ANXIETY THE CURRENT MEDICAL VIEW 104
- CHAPTER 20: NLP HACKS TO REPLACE ANXIETY WITH HAPPINESS 115
- CHAPTER 21: IMPROVE YOUR CONCENTRATION 119
- CHAPTER 22: THE POWER OF POSITIVE THINKING......... 130
- CHAPTER 23: MINDFULNESS MEDITATION 132
- CHAPTER 24: RECOVERING AND REDISCOVERING 135
- CHAPTER 25: BODY SCAN MEDITATION- WHY DO IT AND HOW TO DO IT... 150
- CHAPTER 26: INTERNAL STRESSORS 156
- CHAPTER 27: MEDITATE FOR PERSONAL DISCOVERY 165
- CHAPTER 28: SECTION SEVEN... 175
- CHAPTER 29: HOW TO SLEEP WELL AGAIN 183

Introduction

In this day and age where lives have become extremely hectic, everybody needs a release that can help them stave off illnesses that are not only physical in nature but also mental.

Unlike physical illnesses, mental illnesses are difficult to cure, as they vary greatly from person to person, and do not come with a single type of treatment. Some of these include stress, anxiety and extreme anger.

If you happen to suffer from any of these and would like to find a solution to your problem, then you have come to the right place! This book will act as your guide to meditation and usher your life in the right direction.

You will learn how meditation can help you combat stress, anxiety and anger and to lead a happy life.

I hope you have a good time reading this book!

Chapter 1: Evaluate What You Lose When You Fail To Defy Your Shyness

The first question you should ask yourself is why bother to do something about your shyness? What do you lose when you fail to voice your opinions and become more adventurous? We are going to start our discussion by looking at what you stand to lose by not trying to build your confidence

Life Changing Opportunities

One of the greatest losses you will experience because of your introverted nature is the loss of several opportunities that would have changed your life forever. Each time your shyness keeps you away from attending a business meeting or meeting someone new, you have lost the chance to learn something that could have altered the course of your life and channeled you towards a more productive life.

Think about all those times you failed to talk to somebody about your business plans. Think about the times that you missed talking to someone you loved because you could not make the first move. Think about all the times you passed a speaking opportunity to someone else.

All these lost opportunities could have changed your life. While you may have lost several of such opportunities in the past, more are in the future; the only way to ensure you do not lose the future ones is to substitute your shyness with confidence beginning today.

Beautiful Relationships

Another important thing you lose to shyness is the chance to enjoy beautiful relationships that would have possibly led to marriage. Shy people easily give up on the love of their lives and end up with people not good enough for them. This happens because shyness keeps one from voicing his or her intentions to the ones he or she truly loves.

Recall the number of times you have missed the chance to settle down with someone amazing; this is an indicator of what you lose to shyness. Addressing the issue of your shyness will help you meet someone special and enjoy a rewarding relationship.

The Chance to Maximize Your Potential

When you are too shy to go out to where things are happening and where you will be easy to notice, you lose the chance to attain the zenith of your career.

Shyness keeps you from being daring enough to venture into new business opportunities and stops you from attempting great feats. Shyness stops you from being bold enough to try what most people tried and failed. Shyness stops you from trying to stand out from the crowd. Most people you see as celebrities today are not 'touched' by God; they just boldly pursued their dreams.

So, shyness will definitely make you lose a lot in life but what do you do?

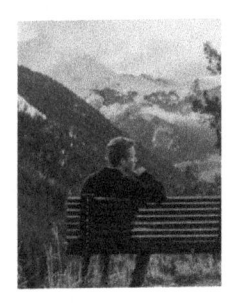

Chapter 2: Intermediate techniques

Remember that this isn't like a sport, where you need to do more in a shorter span of time. Mindfulness is always with you and you can take it with you wherever you go because it's an understanding of what's happening in your own mind. To see the spiritual side of the experience, these techniques help you to appreciate the world around you and to see things that you normally don't give yourself enough time to notice.

Technique Six - Being Inspired

For this exercise chose a place that makes you feel humbled. It could be a beauty spot at sunset or your backyard at sunrise. Whatever area it is, it should be something that awes you. I find the coastline does this but not when it's filled to brimming with people. Thus quiet times are the best. Sit down and breathe as I showed you in Technique One. Keep your back straight. Close your eyes until your breathing has achieved the rhythm that means it is regular and without pauses. Now open your eyes and look at the scene and think of nothing else. See how small you are compared with the beauty that surrounds you. Being humble makes you stronger. It makes you more compassionate and giving because you lose all of those false premises that advertising places on you every day of your life. Be inspired and use all of your senses to enjoy the moment.

Technique Seven - Alternate Breathing

This technique is helpful during the day when you find that you are a little overwhelmed and need a little more energy. Hold your thumb over your right nostril and breathe in deeply through your left nostril. Now switch over to covering the right nostril, while the breath is still inside you and breathe out through the other nostril. When you breathe out using this technique, you need to imagine that you are breathing out all of the bad stuff in your life. It may make a little bit of a noise, so do it somewhere you don't have to stress about it. What this does is help you to clear your mind so that you have more energy and vitality as well as clarity.

Technique Eight - Mindless thought

If you have not yet read the book by Elizabeth Gilbert or seen the movie "Eat, Pray, Love" it's a shame because there is a perfect example of when the character in the story took a trip to an Ashram to get away from the fact that her marriage was falling to pieces. This was a voyage of discovery and her guru asked her and other participants to sit and to clear the mind of thought. She couldn't do it because she felt that her thoughts had more importance than silence.

We often feel like the thoughts are tangible things, but they aren't. In fact, the harder you try not to think, the harder it is to actually blank your mind. This technique is all about sitting and concentrating on something that you find inspires you or that fascinates you and letting go of all other thought. It's like allowing your mind to be present in the moment but not to wander elsewhere. Remember, it's only a technique and you can master it, but you master it best when you don't actually try.

Sit in a comfortable position and breathe as I showed you in Technique one, with your back straight so that the flow of energy goes down through your body and you don't have blocked energy points. At the same time look at something you choose to focus upon. Look at every detail and when you find your mind wandering, pull it back to thinking about that object you chose. For example, if you are looking at a leaf, imagine the texture from what you see. What would it be like to touch it? What color is it? Do the colors change with the light? Can you see the veins in the leaf? Look deeper than you have ever looked at something before and at the same time keep the same rhythm of breathing going.

Sometimes you feel like this after you have just watched a great movie and there are still fragments of the story in your mind. This technique helps you to get rid of negative thinking and replace it with something more tangible that you can hold onto, enjoying whatever it is that you chose as your focal point. It's like looking at the same world though from an optimistic viewpoint rather than a pessimistic point of view.

Chapter 3: Step 1: Determine Whether You Have An Anxiety Disorder

One way of determining whether you have anxiety or not is by looking out for the symptoms. Unfortunately, the symptoms of anxiety disorders are also symptoms of a thousand and one more conditions. This makes it impossible for you to be 100% sure that the reason behind the symptoms you are experiencing is actually an anxiety disorder. After the following symptoms therefore, I will expound some more with situations, which can help you know better whether or not what you are experiencing are actually signs of anxiety disorders or hopefully something milder.

Lack of emotion where you appear to have your emotions' valve turned off because you cannot feel anything despite the situation.

Paranoia about people's thoughts where you are always convinced that people do not think positively about you and that they hate you etc.

Feelings of depression, which just pop up from nowhere and for no particular reason.

A sense of impending doom, which results from no particular trigger but you just feel as if something terrible is about to happen to you or those close to you.

Trembling, which you cannot stop and which has no trigger whatsoever.

Feeling panicked yet there are no rational triggers of the panic.

Feeling tired more often than not even when nothing draining or difficult has been done and the feeling is continuous.

Failure to think of anything other than the current worry no matter how you try. You still find your mind going back to the worry as much as you try to think about some other things.

Irritability in situations and incidences that you would ordinarily not be irritated in or about

Blurred vision that just comes without any warning and without any trigger

Feeling as if you are going crazy because all kinds of thoughts are whirling around in your head. You also feel as if people are looking at you as if you are going crazy.

Lack of sleep where you toss and turn and worry about something that should never give you sleepless nights.

Long lasting disturbing thoughts, which you can't seem to shake off no matter what you do or how hard you try.

Continuous nightmares especially about things that happened to you or that you witnessed even several years after the experience.

A racing heart that just starts with no particular trigger and this becomes a constant occurrence

Feelings of powerlessness that make you dejected because you see yourself unable to do anything to help yourself

Feelings of hopelessness that drive you into feeling so sorry for yourself that you even contemplate suicide as a good option

Headaches, which are so serious that you can't think, especially making you feel as if you have a tight band around your head.

Excessive sweating especially from under your feet, in your palms and arm pits yet there is no real reason why you should be sweating that much.

You can agree with me though that the above symptoms can mean something yet they can also mean nothing.

The following is a list of anxiety disorders risk factors, which when coupled with the symptoms might lead to a better but still not final conclusion.

If you are someone with an inclination to negativity or a timid temperament, you might be more prone to anxiety disorders.

If someone in your family suffers from or suffered from an anxiety disorder, then you might be at risk.

If you are female, you might be at risk as more women are affected by anxiety disorders twice more than men except in the case of obsessive-compulsive disorder.

Age can have an effect on panic disorders normally occurring in teenage years while separation anxiety mostly happens in early childhood.

Traumatic experiences at a certain point in your life can lead to a higher risk of anxiety disorders.

If you abuse alcohol and drugs and if you drink too much caffeinated drinks, you could be at a higher risk than most people.

Although the points above might not be conclusive on whether you have an anxiety disorder, they can be a good starting point to help you determine if you could be having a problem. Knowing the different types of anxiety will probably make it a lot easier to truly understand that you have anxiety after knowing some of more general symptoms associated with anxiety. However, before we get to that, you should learn about the indicators that you truly need to do something about the situation.

Chapter 4: Social Anxiety

It is normal for most of us to feel anxious when we need to speak in a group or when we meet someone for the first time. Yet, there are countless simple situations like these that can result in such anxious moments for some people that it cripples their day to day life. Society anxiety is nothing but fear of handling social situations, no matter how small they are. Here are some signs of social anxiety:

- Always being worried about how others will react
- Being extremely nervous when participating in social situations
- Feeling highly insecure about everything you do or say in a social situation
- A sense of paranoia
- Feeling that everybody is judging you
- Avoiding social gatherings completely
- Physical symptoms such as increased heart rate, rapid breathing, sweating, etc.

- Avoiding eye contact

Tips to Overcome Social Anxiety

Share Your Problem – Suppressing or hiding anxiety will only compound the problem. The first and, perhaps, the most effective step to take is to share your fears with people. You could choose someone you trust or approach an online support group. It is common for many people to think that sharing such problems will make them a butt of social jokes as society, even today, frowns down on any form of mental weakness. Remember that all of us need help and it requires courage to seek help. Go seek help and benefit yourself and others as well.

Breathe – The human body is very powerful. It has some amazing ways of healing itself. First, identify signs of anxiety. For some, it could be the stiffening of the body. For others, it could be excessive sweating. Find out yours. Your body and especially your lungs will help you alleviate these symptoms.

Breathing exercises work wonderfully in these situations. When you focus on steadying your breath, it has a direct effect on the heart rate, which will slow down gradually. When your heart rate slows down, your mind and thoughts will also have reduced agitation thereby helping you relax and overcome the anxious moments.

Thoughts Are Not Real – No matter how seemingly powerful anxiety is, you must will yourself to remember that these are mere thoughts and they are not real. You control your reality. Social anxiety feeds on negative thoughts and unduly emphasizes on non-existent danger. Sweating and increased heart rates are results of these thoughts only.

Fortunately, creating thoughts is a habit and you can always change the habit for more positive results than before. The cure for anxiety is not merely positivity but also realistic thinking. Examine your anxious thoughts which might be saying, "Now I'm going to say something stupid and make a fool of myself." Look at these and remind yourself that they are exaggerations of reality. Now, try and create thoughts that are more realistic and calm your anxiety away.

Refocus Your Attention – Anxious moments are very powerful to grab your full attention so much so that they make you turn your focus inwards without you even realizing it. Suddenly, you will begin to notice your heartbeat increasing, you are getting red in the face, you are sweating, etc. These attention-grabbing tactics seem to take on a domino effect as they rapidly pass onto the next making you forget the external world.

Be aware of this and refocus your attention. If you are in the midst of talking to someone when this is happening, focus on the conversation minutely. If you are doing some task, bring your focus to the task at hand. Don't internalize the anxious moments. Throw them off gear by shifting your attention to other things around you.

Don't be Afraid to Face Your Fears – The biggest mistake you can do when it comes to overcoming social anxiety is avoiding social situations. While this might give you temporary reprieve, it prevents you from learning how to cope. The more you avoid, the less equipped you become at managing these situations and the more intense your fears will become.

Instead, face your fears. Initially, take the help of a trusted friend. Go to a party with the friend and use him or her as a shield to start conversations. Then, make the attempt to talk to strangers; people you are certain you will not meet again. Start confidently and slowly. But don't run away. Running away will give you the same result and zero learning. Staying and facing your fears will give you opportunities you didn't know existed.

Avoid Perfectionism – Today's world is seemingly trying to achieve the elusive perfection. The social media platforms and the images posted there appear to reflect a life of absolute harmony and no discord at all. Remember this is far, far from the truth for everyone on this earth. Everyone is fighting his or her own battles and failing more often than winning.

Avoid trying to be perfect. You are wasting valuable resources on an unattainable status instead of using those resources to make yourself a better person today than you were yesterday. Making mistakes enhances our learning in ways that successes can never match up to.

Get Used to Rejections in a Slow Manner – Treat it like a game and move level by level. Here are some challenges you can put for yourself at different levels:

Beginner Level

- Ask a stranger for the time

- Give someone a compliment

- Start a conversation with someone outside the set of people you know

- Put your hand up to answer a question. Keep an answer ready if you are called. It needn't be something related to the subject. You could simply stand up and say, "Sorry ma'am, I misunderstood the question. I don't know the answer to this." Remember you are not trying to get the right answer. You are only trying to overcome social anxiety

Intermediate Level

●At the billing, ask for a discount

●Request someone to take a snap of you

●Ask the strictest teacher in your class for an extension to do your assignment. It doesn't matter if you have already finished. Just go and ask.

●Talk to a friend with whom you fought and try and make up with him or her

●In a line, ask if you can go in front

●Help in fundraising for a charity that you believe in

Advanced Level

●Dance in public

- Speak to a set of new people sitting together in a group at a social event

Social anxiety is the most common type. Just remember you are not alone and there are many out there in the world who are struggling with the same problem. If you feel that you are unable to control your anxiety, do not hesitate to approach a professional for help.

Chapter 5: Why Should You Spend Your Time to Read All These Pages?

Before you start reading you should know why this content is written. The content has been written with an intention to provide you the best solution to manage your anxiety. Yes, I am talking about "Anxiety" you are facing every day in your life. Actually anxiety arises from your mind and also solution of anxiety is hidden in your mind. But you don't know how to control your mind and the resulting anxiety. In your daily life your mind alters and you become anxious due to various reasons. These reasons may be personal, social, official or even it may arise due to your poor health condition. Whatever the reasons are, anxiety sufferers face a lot of troubles in their life. Sufferers may lose their mental peace and happiness due to anxiety. The mental unrest due to anxiety hampers their normal life. They become irritated with simple change of environment around them. Even at favourable environment they suffer greatly from their fear.

Nowadays anxiety and meditation are widely uttered terms among the sufferers. There are lot of queries:

What is anxiety?

What are the effects of anxiety?

Is meditation worthy to relieve anxiety?

How can I perform meditation?

What is the best meditation practice?

How long should I meditate?

How many times in a day I need to meditate?

What are the requirements for performing meditation?

These are the common queries everybody wants to know. I can make sure that you will get all the answers here. Just spend some of your time to read this book. You will get all the answers and you will find the solution to get relief from anxiety.

Here I have tried to elaborate the term "Anxiety". For your better understanding I have written about its origin, its nature and about its common symptoms. You should know the vulnerability caused by anxiety. By reading the content you will know how anxiety can hamper your mental and physical condition.

Many times you have listened about meditation from your family, friends and even from the media. But the true fact is that all the times you have received incomplete information. You may hear that meditation is really effective in relieving anxiety. But you didn't hear how to perform it, when to perform it, and how long to perform it. What is the right way? Then this book will provide you the necessary information to perform your mediation perfectly. From here you will learn about the best meditative practice and the way you should meditate.

Breathing meditation is one of the most popular forms among different meditation practices due its simplicity and effectiveness. From your reading you will get the information about how to perform breathing meditation and its effectiveness on relieving anxiety.

The purpose of this book is to provide you the information about the common causes of anxiety and how to manage anxiety by meditation. There are different types of meditation, defined and used for specific purposes. I have tried to describe the functions of breathing meditation in controlling anxiety. With the help of this book you will know how to control your mind and get relief from anxiety. Here we are giving emphasize on breathing meditation as it is the easiest one with very high benefits. Meditation is simple practice which you can perform easily in your everyday life. Different professionals can do it regularly spending few minutes in a day. By continuing breathing meditation, you will get rid of anxiety from your life. You will get the ability to control your mind and will get inner peace.

Therefore, I am requesting your attention before you start reading the content. I am not claiming that this book will change your life but after reading all these contents you will be able to change your life.

Chapter 6: Depression and its complications

Depression is one of the most common mental disorders that can either strike abruptly or be extremely long term. A common misconception regarding depression is that depression is not actually a disorder and is instead regarded as "feeling down" and thus can be easily overcome through force of will. Regrettably, this is the result of the word "depressed" being used too often and is far from the truth. Therefore, people who suffer from depression are likely to feel isolated as it can be hard to difficult to find others who can relate to their circumstance. In fact depression is considered to be the leading cause of disability worldwide.

As many of those reading this book may be familiar with, depression is very serious and is synonymous with a host of negative conditions such as:

Lethargy

Feelings of hopelessness, emptiness, sadness, guilt and lack of self-worth

Apathy

Insomnia and disturbed sleep

Appetite loss

Irritability

Thoughts of suicide

And the list goes on…

Ultimately, the types of symptoms are the same amongst the many types of depression though the number of symptoms and combinations may differ from individual to individual.

So just where do we begin in curing depression?By believing it's possible!Yes I know it sounds immensely clichébut the sad fact is that many believe that their condition is impossible to cure. Many professionals agree that some of the top causes of depression stem from:

Brain chemistry imbalances

It has been noted that abnormal functioning of brain circuits that regulate emotions and the fight-or-flight system makes a person prone to having depressive disorders

Hormonal fluctuations

Hereditary and genetic causes

Current research into depression suggests a strong link between genetics and depression. Statistics show that there is a higher chance of a person suffering from depression in cases whereby a first-degree relative of the individual has been previously diagnosed with the disorder.

Childhood trauma

Many brain disorders have a strong link with psychological factors. A person may develop depression due to traumatic events that happened in earlier periods of their lives. Embarrassing or humiliating events during childhood (e.g being bullied or neglected) are common events that impact the self-esteem of an individual. This is important as low self-esteem has been shown to be highly correlated with depression and a host of other disorders (e.g social anxiety disorder).

One positive element about the list above is that steps can be taken to rectify everything mentioned besides being born with faulty genetics, which is rare. I stressed at the start of this book that an open mind must be adopted precisely because more than a few people will react negatively to any prospect that suggests that they are in control of their mental health. This is understandable since we are dealing with depression disorder in which negativity and helplessness are part of. Do not forget that the brain has been known to be very plastic and adaptable. Therefore, at least until you have tried tackling your disorder with some of the methods found in this book and elsewhere; discount the possibility that your body was not born with the disorder but instead the depression was brought about by environmental factors.

The perspective that depression is a disease in which one has no control over how their body functions is harmful and is an unhealthy mentality that will be detrimental to ones efforts. Most of the time, (except in rare circumstances) the affected individual is **not** born with dysfunctional dopamine receptors (this will be explained in chapter 2) and does possess vast potential to alleviate themselves of depression. As such, I will require you to believe that treating depression naturally is possible.

Be aware that many uninformed doctors are quick to resort to prescribing drugs to combat depression. Many of these drugs can have negative side effects with the additional downside that the body can develop dependency on them.

Even if a professional diagnosed you with the disorder and even if your family has a history clinical depression, believe that you can be cured for now and follow the rest of the steps in the book. After all you stand very little to lose and have everything to gain.

With that in mind, let us move into chapter 2 in which we will be attempting to treat depression from a biological perspective.

Chapter 7: Acceptance

Acceptance is not giving in. We are NOT giving in to anxiety. We are just merely accepting that it is a part of who we are and letting go of the hate we have against it. When you constantly fight anxiety, you are feeding it more energy. You are giving it more power and more control. When you stop fighting and accept it for what it is, you regain control. It becomes less powerful over you and a lot less intimidating.

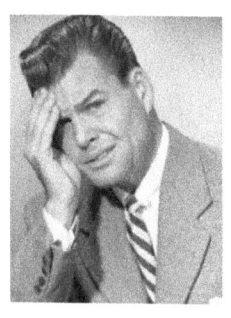

I'm sorry...

You want me to do

WHAT

with my anxiety?

You know what? Anxiety is the most common form of mental illness and its estimated that approximately 10 percent of teenagers and 40 percent of adults suffer from an anxiety disorder of some kind. So, although it feels like it, you're most definitely not alone! You are absolutely and undeniably surrounded by people who feel just like you do. The issue is, many times we are unaware of this since we treat it like some sort of horrible, shameful secret and so we live in our tiny little bubbles thinking no one understands or cares to understand.

Only those who I was very close with knew about my anxiety disorder. Very few knew I took medication for it and even fewer knew how greatly it had negatively impacted my life. Chronic anxiety can be a very lonely and painful way to live as most of our time is spent inside of our own heads. While it wasn't easy at first, and still to this day can be a tough topic to bring up with some, once I decided I was no longer going to feel ashamed for something I didn't voluntarily choose to live with and started to openly discuss it with friends and even strangers, it not only

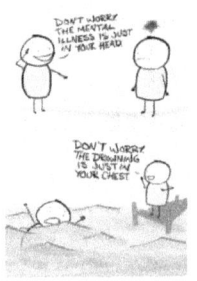

eased my anxiety but opened up a whole new world for me.

You see, the worry of judgement and ridicule only feeds the anxiety. It just gives you more to be anxious about. Letting go of those worries **eases** anxiety. Some aren't going to understand what you're going through and that's ok. Some may judge or simply tell you "it's all in your head" but that's ok too because those who are ignorant to what anxiety is will be out numbered by those who are going to turn to you and say, "No, way?! Me too!" There will also be those who have never experienced it but will be supportive because they care about you. You may also be surprised to find that many of your friends and family will educate themselves on the subject just to be a better support system for you.

If you cannot accept yourself for who you are, how can anyone else? You set the stage, this is your life and if you can stand up for yourself and all that you are, flaws and all, the world is only going to see you as a stronger human being for doing so.

Accepting my anxiety and letting go of the shame and embarrassment I had towards myself for having anxiety disorder was the first and by far the most significant step in taking back my control.

Chapter 8: Using a Mantra

If you find your mind wandering when you count your breaths, here's another simple (and classic) method. Just like the Zen technique mentioned earlier, it involves distracting your mind. But unlike the Zen method, a mantra works on several levels. It can be sung like a Gregorian chant. Using consonants to vibrate as you sing. It can be said aloud, or repeated quietly to yourself. All methods involve letting your mind focus on the mantra, which has little or no meaning to ponder. The mind settles into simple repetition and quiets itself.

The simple silent method only involves choosing a word or phrase to repeat to yourself. Some popular English choices are Home, Silent, Goodnight, and Sunshine. Simply repeat the word you choose over and over to yourself. Do it in a comfortable position for twenty minutes, if you have time. You'll find the word loses meaning as you repeat it. Your breathing will slow, and your body will deeply relax.

Non-English words work just efficiently. "OM" is a world favorite. Take a deep breath, then release it slowly as you think the mantra to yourself. The word can also be hummed softly. The "m" vibrates as it is hummed, causing a calming effect. After about twenty minutes, you'll feel calm and even a bit spacey. Take a few deep breaths and allow yourself to "come back" before standing up, or you may feel dizzy.

You can use a mantra when exercising as well. You won't feel relaxed physically, but your mind will center and stop the mental "chatter." Phrases tend to work well while jogging, walking, or riding a bicycle. "Stronger and Stronger" works well for many people. You can choose your own, or use a simpler single term, like "Sunshine" or "Tomorrow."

Whatever mantra you choose, the effect is to let the mind focus on one word or phrase that allows it to stop worrying and jabbering about daily concerns. When it quiets, the mind's interference is silent, allowing for moments of insight or inspiration to slip through. When you "return" from meditating, you may find solutions to problems or original ideas have popped into your head. Or, you may simply feel relaxed and centered. That alone is fine!

Organized meditation schools often assign a mantra to students. The student does not know what their mantra means. But when the mantra is practiced twice a day, breathing slows and relaxation grows. The Transcendental Meditation (TM) school has studies that measure the beneficial results (www.tm.org). Their program costs money, but for people who want scientific evidence before they try meditating, it's worth a look. Many other schools of meditation involve religious beliefs, but the basic techniques are the ones described above.

Another simple technique for beginners involves no mantra but is a simple breathing exercise. In a quiet space where you can relax, begin to breathe slowly and deeply. As you do, picture the breath you inhale as a golden mist. Fee; it is filling your lungs, full of health and freshness. Then as you exhale, imagine a gray mist full of unwanted thoughts and negative feelings. With every breath you inhale, you fill yourself with health, energy, and calm. With each gray mist you exhale, you will rid yourself of tension and negative stress. In fifteen minutes, you will feel like a new, healthy person.

It may seem hard to accept that such a simple exercise can alter your physical being. But the images you project can significantly affect you. Here's a simple demonstration of how we can energize each other.

With a group of four people, choose one to direct and one to be the subject, Have the subject leave the room for a few minutes. The director then tells the others that when he says "RED" they should stare at the subject and visualize the subject as ill, coughing, and exhausted. At that point, the director should ask the subject to hold out an arm and keep it stiff. The subject will hold it out, and the director will push down on it. There will be little resistance.

Then the group should learn that when the Director says "GREEN," they should see the subject as full of health and energy. The subject should seem as if he or she is tan and ready to exercise. When the group is told "GREEN," they should stare accordingly, with the director. The subject will hold out an arm that will not budge. The difference will be noticeable. The subject will also feel wonderful, just as you will after breathing in the gold mist. Be sure to leave the subject with the "GREEN" condition.

It may seem like a simple exercise, but it works and shows us the power of visualization. The golden mist will invigorate you. The gray mist will leave you feeling clean. And the steady breathing will have the meditative effect you're after.

Chapter 9: Therapies

Cognitive behavioral therapy

There are several ways of curing anxiety and panic attacks that lead to control of stress and depression. The first method involves cognitive behavioral therapy. This method is the most effective way of controlling anxiety and panic attacks and finally eliminating them. It focuses on thinking patterns and behaviors that trigger the attacks. It helps look at fears in a more realistic angle. It raises the question 'What is the worst that can happen in the given situation?' Hence, you get to learn that nothing disastrous can happen as a result of the situation. Also, all emotions even the most crippling fears that may lead to great anxiety or panic attacks are temporary, they come and go and cannot get a long lasting grip on you. If you keep this in mind, the intensity of panic attacks will be significantly reduced.

Cognitive therapy sessions by highly trained professionals are highly recommended for individuals with extreme cases. They may have some financial implications but are most effective in getting rid of the attacks completely.

Relaxation therapy

Relaxation techniques are also very helpful in dealing with anxiety, stress and depression. They include meditation, yoga, autogenic training, Qigong, self-hypnosis, mind-body relaxation, deep breathing, visualization and massage. They are not only fun but also relaxing and can make a very big difference. They are highly recommended to those with severe anxiety and stress. They elevate feel good hormones such as serotonin and reduce stress hormones. In addition, they improve your overall health enabling your body to deal with stressful events therefore preventing panic attacks. The techniques also help with cardiac health, immune system support, stress management, anger management, headache, high blood pressure, pain management, addiction treatment and insomnia hence it is a solution to a multiple of problems you may be experiencing. Some of the techniques may require guidance by experts therefore having some financial implications but they are easy to learn. You can attend one or two sessions and learn to conduct your own sessions at the comfort of your living room. The steps are also available in various resource books, websites and YouTube hence you can easily get the content. However, it is important to note that different situations are dealt with a specific technique and the choice depends on other factors such as an individual's fitness level therefore it is important to consult the experts so that they recommend one for you in order to attain optimum results.

Chapter 10: So, what's the secret ingredient?

Achieving positive mental health is not as tough as you might think. Of course, if you're going to view it as a task or a chore, it's bound to get tiring.

You're thus far into the book and you've yet to find out what's the secret ingredient. Voila! You're the secret ingredient.

Cliche, I know, but bear with me and give me a chance.

From this part of the book, you need to keep in mind these two very important things. Effort and mindset. One cannot magically achieve positive mental health as if you're buying groceries from amazon prime.

You can't get it with one day shipping. It's a process. It's a mental effort from yourself. You have to make a conscious effort to want to be mentally healthy.

On top of that, you have to actively take steps in the right direction.

For one, you bought this book and you made it this far, so kudos to you!

Let's talk about having the correct mindset now. To learn how to frame your mind, to slowly reach out of your comfort zone. Surrounding yourself with positivity would naturally make you happier, even if you aren't used to the positive things. That's the end goal for this book. To make you happier.

For instance, if you take pride in brewing your own cup of coffee every morning, why not take an extra second to appreciate the aroma to start your day on a good note?

The better question would be this. What makes you happy? What could be done to make yourself happier? Are you doing it enough? Are you giving yourself enough credit for your achievements? If you've correctly identified what makes you happy, do more of it.

That being said, try to keep it logical and realistic. No big ticket impulse buys for you.

Maybe try being cherrier to your neighbor tomorrow morning, or replacing that old tupperware bottle you have been using forever.

Having an open mind is crucial to being happier. You've got to be open to learning new things. And I don't mean insane stunts like sky-diving or whatnot. I mean small little things, like volunteering at the local soup kitchens, or even trying out the newest flavor of ice cream you've been eyeing. They go hand in hand, but it can be daunting, so best to start small and work your way up.

Chapter 11: How to Combat Anxiety and Avoid Panic Attacks

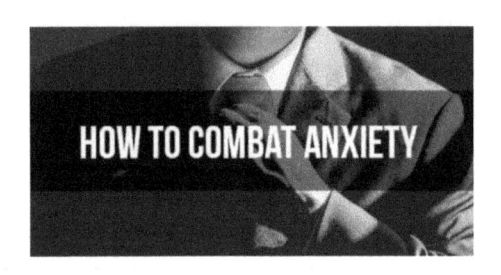

For those who experience panic attacks what can you do to Begin getting back them? There are a number of different options available to you but the aim is to a) get yourself to safety and b) begin to address the symptoms.

Here we will look at how best to manage a situation where you find yourself beginning to suffer from an attack...

Panic Attack Symptoms

Before you can begin to treat a panic attack, you first need to be able to identify the symptoms of one. This will provide you 'early warning' so you can start to put a plan into action that will help yourself to calm down and return to normal function.

The symptoms of a panic attack then comprise:

- Shallow breathing
- Racing, negative thoughts
- Sweating
- Muscle tension
- Dizziness
- Chest pain
- Pacing

Often the heart rate where it is so extreme that it can reach the point feels like you are having a heart attack. This is one of the problems people face when suffering from panic attacks: they become convinced that they are currently suffering!

The symptoms take about 10-20 minutes to reach their peak and will often subside but sometimes take a few hours. Of course it is important to get if you think yourself checked. There is any possibility that you may be experiencing a heart attack.

Note that in cases of heart attack the feeling of dread will tend to precede the heart rate or the stress. Panic attacks also cause restlessness vibration, rapid and shallow the best way is turned up to 11 although as being like a flight or fight response.

In case you've ever had to give a speech in public that you've been scared to give, if you've ever had a confrontation with someone in the street, or if you've ever gotten into a serious argument with someone in a shop, then you will likely have experienced these symptoms.

This is with the added breathing issues and dizziness and what a panic attack feels like but a little worse. If that's what you are experiencing, then you are probably suffering with not a heart attack and a panic attack.

You can be sure of the actually but, if you are ever uncertain then it's always worth speaking with your GP to be on the safe side. Consider as well the aspect of risk factors and demographics.

Heart

The next way to tell the difference between panic attack or heart attack Is to examine the nature of the torso pain. It's the chest pain that makes us suspect we're having a heart attack when it's 'just' a panic attack.

The chest pain is quite different. At a heart attack for example, the pain is described as a 'crushing' pain and a dull ache, like somebody is sitting on your chest causing a shortness of breath. In a panic attack the difficulty breathing Is Really caused By hyperventilation rather than heart issues and this will be experienced as CO_2 and dizziness rather than a feeling as if you're about to suffocate. Any 'tightness' will be caused by muscle contractions which are caused by stress.

What is a Normal Heart Rate during a Panic Attack?

Seeing as anxiety increases your heart rate (through adrenaline) and panic Attacks are stress episodes, it makes sense that your heart rate should increase at this time. But what is a normal panic attack heartbeat? Unfortunately, the answer is not straight forward.

For starters, everyone has a different resting heart rate with meaning they start from base-lines that are different to begin. An athlete may have a resting heart rate as low as 40bpm or less, whereas someone unhealthy may have a heart rate as large as 120bpm when they are not doing anything. Heart rate is dictated by Fitness because exercise to a large extent the more powerful the heart becomes as a muscle, the more it will have the ability to drive blood.

This means that a heart will not have to beat to be able to circulate as blood. Other factors affect heart rate however, include blood viscosity and vasodilation, metabolism height and more. The air temperature can impact your heart rate.

Some people have heart rates for reason. A panic attack heart rate then is likely to result in a marked and sudden spike for that individual it might still be beating at slower than some people not having a panic attack.

As a general rule though, you can expect a panic attack heart Rate to be anything from 100 to 170bpm equivalent to an intensive bout of exercise. What's also important to keep in mind though, is that everyone experiences panic attacks and every case of a panic attack is different.

Managing Anxiety and Panic Attacks

In the short term, there are a few things you can do to help manage the Symptoms of a panic attack and also to get yourself back to safety and under control.

Get to Safety

The first and most important thing is to get yourself to safety. Panic attacks cause disassociation headedness and hyperventilation. There is a real danger of falling over or having an accident if you're in control of a vehicle.

For all these reasons, you should try to get to safety if you notice the signs of a panic attack beginning to set in and that way you can make certain that you won't be likely to fall over or to crash a vehicle.

If you are in public, tell someone how you're feeling and find a spot where you can breathe to sit down. Then calmly take another chance to pull over if you are driving.

Treat Hyperventilation

Chance that you might be suffering with hyperventilation. This occurs when we get overexcited which in turn leads to us consequently lowering CO_2 and breathing quickly.

This is the reason why they can even make you fall over or pass out and that anxiety attacks will lead to feelings of light-headedness and dizziness. These all can give you ideas of what to do to help get your breathing back in order.

Breathe Slowly

With or without hyperventilation, it's important to get your breathing under to make a conscious effort to try to breathe slowly and deeply and control. This is one of the main methods advocated by cognitive therapists as a way to stop the anxiety attack symptoms and to help restore order. Breathing deeply and slowly is effective because it promotes the Activation of the 'parasympathetic nervous system'.

This is the system within the body that acts against the sympathetic nervous system and which puts the body in a restful 'rest and digest state' that is essentially the opposite of the fight or flight reaction.

Breathe Into a Bag

Panic attacks Provide Start breathing faster and faster to the point where you upset the balance of carbon dioxide in your blood. In other words -- too much CO_2 and not enough O_2.

The remedy is to breathe into a bag which forces you to 'rebreathe' the air adjusting the balance back to levels that are healthy and normal. You might find that using some form of medicine or as mentioned maybe essential oils can be beneficial for treating symptoms.

Then this is a fantastic way to decrease the symptoms if you really can't afford to get an attack. Over time, however, the objective is to utilize the skills taught in another section to prevent needing medication in any respect.

Calm Your Thoughts

When we have panic attacks, they will often occur alongside anxious these and thoughts could include fears of death. As previously mentioned, these rumination's are both signs of panic attacks and causative factors creating a vicious cycle. Key in recovering from panic attacks then is to try to keep calm.

This In turn means being disciplined with your ideas and using positive affirmations etc. to attempt to reassure yourself that nothing bad is going to happen. You can learn thought techniques designed to help you combat panic by seeing a cognitive therapist strikes.

These are therapists that provide thinking tools which can enable you to know what to do during a panic in addition to during responses and in many of other situations. Try to remind yourself that the best course of action is to allow the attack run its course. Provided that you are sitting down and you are safe, no threat is posed by a panic attack and is nothing to be embarrassed about.

So the best thing you can actually do? That is to simply act normal. And it's practicing this ability to act normal that will help You to reduce the occurrence of panic attacks in the long-term...

How to Combat Anxiety and Panic Attacks by Controlling Your Thoughts and Emotions

First place? The answer relates back to what we have learned about neurotransmitters

And hormones in previous chapters. When our brain 'does something' an action potential fires causing electricity to nip along our neurons. This in turn releases a number and whether or not the encounter should be cemented by us.

In other words then, it is connection and the formation of specific neurons, releasing certain neurotransmitters which lead to panic and anxiety attacks. And this web of interconnected neurons is formed by our experiences and our thought processes -- resulting in what is known as a 'connectome'.

The point is that it's all going on 'in your head'. It is all to do with the way that information has been encoded by your mind and it is all to do with the way that you perceive what's currently happening. In other words, if you see a lion but you think it is a cat, then you will produce oxytocin rather than adrenaline (and you will die). If a deadline is seen by you and believe you can make it just fine, then you will produce serotonin rather than cortisol. It's not actually the danger which is causing you to have the panic attack, it's your perception of risk.

And for some of us, our perception is not a fair and completely skewed reflection of the reality. This is the reason some people end up with phobias and anxiety disorders. And in the case of panic attacks, this is related to phobias or agoraphobia. You feel corners, you feel exposed, you're feeling jostled... and this makes you over-react into the situation. Throw in your reaction to the experience of the panic attack itself and you may wind up working up yourself to the point of passing out. That's a panic attack in a nutshell!

The good news is by changing the way you that you rewire your mind think about things and this means you have neuronal patterns which discharge hormones that are positive than negative ones.

The problem is, that when you have a brain that swimming with stress hormones, making it to form those beliefs that will help to combat stress and difficult for you to think positive about things. Thus you want to use mental discipline so as to help yourself overcome that stress.

The AWARE Technique for Panic Attacks

Mental discipline means reminding yourself constantly that what you're experiencing isn't as bad as you think it is. Or that at least, presuming it is bad will only make matters worse.

For treating anxiety and panic attacks.

A: Accept the anxiety and don't try to fight it.

W: Watch the anxiety as If you were an observer.

A: Act normal.

R: Repeat the other steps.

E: Expect the best. 'Feel' it start to work.

This is essentially a top-down approach that helps you to space yourself in the anxiety by intellectualizing it. By acting normal and going about your usual business, you can teach yourself that a panic attack isn't a huge deal. And the earlier you do this, the sooner you can start to relax and put yourself at ease. Another strategy is one taught in cognitive treatment which

Involves looking at the things you are scared of that led to the panic and anxiety attacks and then assessing whether they are fears that are logical. Can you really get a heart attack? Will people really laugh at you if you faint?

Again, this forces you to think about what's happening and, logically to change the way you respond to stressors. Similarly you can think about the things that led to the anxiety in the first place otherwise. Are you really like if you are late for work to be fired? Is there actually any reason to get stressed when you cannot do anything about it?

We'll talk far more about CBT in the next chapter of this book...

Attacks become less severe and less frequent.

Exposure Therapy

Another kind attacks is exposure therapy. This is a kind of therapy often utilised in the treatment of phobias and involves exposing the person to the thing they are afraid of in conditions so that they know there is no reason to be fearful of them.

Exposure therapy can be helpful for treating anxiety attacks. Here, it is employed by the individual allowing themselves to experience the symptoms of a panic attack once again in a controlled setting. You can become familiar and you can learn how to distinguish them from other ailments or heart attacks. What is more, you will slowly learn that panic attacks in themselves aren't dangerous and while they might be uncomfortable, they don't generally lead to any consequences.

Provided that you are able to sit somewhere, they pass and really there's nothing to be afraid of. Note that exposure therapy here can be used to fight phobias, if phobias are what are causing the anxiety attacks which may be especially useful. As an example, in case you've got a phobia of crowds and this is causing anxiety attacks exposing yourself under controlled conditions to bigger and bigger crowds is a good strategy for coping.

Chapter 12: Other Alternative Therapies for Anxiety

Because most anxiety-related problems are rooted in the psychological field, individuals can opt to undergo therapy. These involve sessions that can last for several weeks or months. Here, a professional will guide them to understand their condition and they can seek his advice on how to overcome it. Since the condition differs for each patient, these therapy sessions would be personalized to best cater to the needs of a certain patient.

One-on-one sessions can be recommended for patients who want a more personal and intimate experience. On the other hand, family members and other loved ones can also support the individual undergoing therapy for better results. Over the years, many forms of therapy have been applied and used for anxiety patients.

Exposure Therapy

Most people with anxiety problems avoid the factors that trigger negative reactions; hence, one way to resolve the issue is to help these people face their fears. In gradually exposing them to the stimulus, they may eventually think more rationally regarding these factors. This process is known as systematic desensitization. In creating a step-by-step process, the patient will gain confidence and consider the stimulus as less threatening; hence, he can control his panic and anxiety reactions.

For example, for someone who is afraid of cockroaches, he can be initially exposed to the insect. To make the event less terrifying, the cockroach can be placed in a transparent sealed container that is a few meters away from him. As the days pass, the patient may take more steps toward the container. The therapist can also try to talk to the patient and explain how harmless the insect is. Eventually, he may be able to at least touch the sealed container.

Through this method, the patient will feel a sense of control over the situation. As a result, he will find the stimulus to be less frightening and may realize that he can confront this in real life. While it is possible to do exposure therapy alone, one can consider doing this simultaneously with CBT.

Other Forms of Therapy

Aside from CBT and Exposure Therapy, individuals can further supplement their treatment by engaging in other forms of therapy. Hypnosis enables an individual to be in a deep state of relaxation. Here, the therapist can create techniques for the patient to face his fears. Biofeedback lets the patient see the anxiety reactions of his body. He would analyze his heart beat and muscle tension. From there, the therapist can recommend ways for him to control these.

Exercise can also help alleviate stress and anxiety. Even thirty minutes of exercise at least thrice a week can create beneficial improvements in the patient's life. Finally, relaxation techniques like meditation, controlled breathing, and visualization can also help treat anxiety. These aim to reduce anxiety and create a more soothing state for the patient.

Chapter 13: How Anxiety Affirmations Can Alleviate Disorders

Since 1952 when Norman Vincent Peale published the first edition of **The Power of Positive Thinking,** mankind in general has embraced the concept that if you think optimistically about life, good things will happen to you.

Years later, the discussion is fresh again as people trying to overcome anxiety disorders are encouraged to embrace positive affirmations. The theory is to tell yourself that you are great and that nothing bad is going to happen to you and it won't. Tell yourself you are wonderful and worthy and by osmosis, others will recognize your value and show their appreciation.

While the concept of repeating positive phrases to yourself to control your anxiety is recognized as an anxiety coping technique, affirmations are not considered to be an anxiety treatment by themselves.

Instead, they are used in conjunction with other forms of therapy as a coping mechanism to help create a brighter mindset for those suffering from GAD.

Those who favor affirmations believe that these positive sayings, repeated silently or vocally in times of intense stress, help people suffering from anxiety disorders to cope and provide an alternate way of looking at the stressful situation.

Typical affirmations can be as simple as "I'm okay," and "I feel well now," or "I am safe; I do not need to run." They can be grand, such as "I have an awesome life," or humble such as "I am at peace."

At the crux of their effectiveness is the belief that if you repeat these positive messages enough, you will begin to believe them and be less plagued by the negative thoughts that prompt anxiety attacks. They are a simple, grounding mechanism when our thoughts are running wild, bringing us gently back to a safe and happy zone. The science behind the idea is based on the concept of cognitive dissonance. In other words, if you say it, you will start to be it, just as an actor who "plays" being a certain character may find himself feeling like that character in certain circumstances.

Positive affirmations are useful in diminishing our negative thoughts that fuel our anxiety. Because negativity promotes fear, stress and feelings of anxiousness, if it can be replaced with positivity, we are less inclined to experience these harmful emotions and replace them with feelings of contentment, peace and calmness.

Using affirmations as a means of relieving anxiety disorders is most effective if you engage them right at the moment when you feel yourself sinking into negative thinking and becoming anxious. Remind yourself that you are in control of yourself, not your anxiety. Remember to think gratefully of the great things in your life and open your mind to make room for calmness and peace to flood in.

When affirming positive thoughts, use your own words, not those of others, even therapists or close friends. They know the words that may calm them, but only you can understand the message you need to hear.

Your affirmation may be that "I am smart enough to make important decisions," or "my hair enhances my beauty" or even "I have charm and that will see me through this unpleasantness." It should be just what you need to hear, not something that you read that worked for somebody else.

Richard T. Kinnier, C. Hofsess, R. Pongratz and C. Lambert conducted a research project into the impact of positive affirmations on people with anxiety. The results of their work, published in June, 2009 in **Psychology and Psychotherapy: Theory, Research and Practice,** discovered that "affirmations relating to 'not being crazy' in relation to anxiety were effective, as were those reminding the anxiety sufferer that their depression would subside in time.

In addition to composing your own personal affirmation messages most reassuring to you, consider writing them as well as speaking them to yourself. At first it may make you feel awkward, like a child writing lines, but the exercise becomes natural and calm-inducing when it is practiced regularly. Any embarrassment you may feel about writing to yourself or talking to yourself is diminished as soon as you start to feel more in harmony with your world.

If you have severe anxiety, you will need to use your affirmations in conjunction with other forms of treatment such as medication or CBT. When you use affirmations, take the time to slowly breathe in and out as you summon your comfort phrases. As you speak slowly, try to imagine the stress and disorder leaving your body, whispering worries floating out of you like vapors over a foggy meadow.

Both mindfulness and affirmations are tools to lessen the anxiety you feel in the moment, and both by their nature flood you with a feeling of awareness of your body. They remind you of the intimate link between what your brain is doing and what your body is doing, and the interwoven patterns linking the two.

In the next chapter we will take that awareness to the next step in alleviating anxiety, and that is to incorporate more physical exercise into your routine.

Chapter 14: Relaxation Techniques

One of the proven methods of treating anxiety and panic attacks is to use relaxation techniques for to calm the mind and have a clear view of things happening around you. We must remember that anxiety and panic attacks are both results of an over-stressed mind. These are five effective relaxation techniques to help empower you!

Progressive relaxation

This whole concept revolves on the observations of visible physical signs happening to people who experience anxiety and panic attacks. Most of the time people experience these attacks tend to have tensed stiff muscles. Progressive relaxation aims to consciously relax each of the major muscle groups of your body. Through this simple technique, tensed up muscles due to anxiety and panic can be easily relaxed and thus lessen its emotional impact. As one improves on this technique, an anxiety sufferer would be able to relax muscles at will and can easily suppress panic and anxiety attacks most effectively!

Applied relaxation

The applied relaxation is the next weapon in the relaxation technique list. This type of relaxation technique is consciously applying relaxation on various muscle locations in the body. With this technique, you can relax yourself and release the tension brewing from stress at your command. In this type of relaxation method you experience "relaxation mantras" which you recite to induce a relaxed state of mind and body. This technique is a much more advanced type of relaxation method, but its effectiveness is profound and is endorsed by psychiatrists and psychologist alike.

The Autogenic training

This involves the capability of the person to consciously calm their emotional and physical aspects. This training helps the person have control over their emotions, learn to control it consciously and understand the power of one's own will and determination to overcome obstacles in life. It is also the main focus of most motivational and life coaches today.

Meditation

Calming the mind through meditation is one of the most frequent relaxation techniques used for people who suffer with anxiety and panic attacks. There are various forms of meditation which you can use such as Yoga. These methods of calming the brain and releasing any kind of negative stress that is burdening it is the main reason why meditation is among the most recommended relaxing techniques to people suffering from anxiety and panic attacks. Meditation has been one of the oldest forms of psychological balancer in human history and its practice has been well documented for thousands of years. For people suffering from anxiety and panic attacks, attending meditation courses can be a big help to help relieve their minds from and reduce the onset of severe panic attacks.

Cognitive behavior therapy

This is by far the most controversial of all anxiety and panic attack treatments today. Cognitive behavior therapy or **CBT** involves teaching the individual to use his or her mind to understand the causes of behavior and emotion and teaches them how to improve one's life through sheer mental willpower. By accessing the mind, the patients can take hold of their emotions by consciously suppressing unwanted emotions by thinking of ways how such emotions are not needed for survival. This method is based on the concept that the mind alone can dictate a person's course of action.

Application of these relaxing techniques

It is important to ensure that all of these 5 relaxing techniques are used properly to regain one's emotional hold in life again.

Make sure that progressive and applied relaxation techniques are done regularly.

This means that you will need to schedule regular relaxing exercise every day. Make sure that every major muscle group is exercised first before you start the relaxation process.

After exercise, begin to relax. Imagine that you are flushing away every burdening stress in your entire body. Each muscle group is relaxed and your whole being is nearing a point of complete relaxation. This can last up to 5 to 15 minutes, depending on your schedule. You can do this lying down or in a seated position; but the main thing is that you should be in a comfortable state of mind to start with.

Once you are in total relaxation begin to meditate. Allow your mind to continuously become active in relaxing your entire body. Visualize anxiety and panic as an object which that you MUST throw away! Like a rock you throw into the lake, each stone you throw into the water signifies a part of your problem leaving you forever!

Finally after meditation, slowly shift your focus into doing productive things immediately. And be sure to rid yourself of any "stinking thinking" for the rest of your day!

Chapter 15: Let's get started

Now you have everything you need to know to start meditating: the place for meditation in a quiet and calm place, the time frame in which you will mediate and the information about the needed posture. You don't need any special pants or sweat tops, no fancy shoes or socks, just wear something that you will be comfortable in – some old sweatpants and washed-out T-shirt, and a cardigan or a hoodie if you normally feel cold. I hope you already set a goal for how long would you be meditating each day. Now we can really start with the practice.

I am inviting you to sit in a comfortable position in the spot of your choice. Turn off your mobile phone or switch to airplane mode and set the alarm to 15 minutes from now.

Relax your whole body with a few deeeeeeep really slow breaths. After you've done so, slowly and attentively close your eyes. Make sure to keep your eyes closed through the entire exercise. That's how you'll get rid off all the distractions on the visual channel.

It is advised that you are breathing through your nose all the time. Inhale through the nose and exhale through the nose. The breathing now should be slowing down, easily coming to its normal natural rhythm. Normal, natural rhythm is allowing you to relax even more. As your rhythm of breathing becomes normal pay slight attention to the pace of the breath and don't try to control it. Any kind of rhythm it may be is perfectly all right. If the breathing is deep, it is deep, and if it is shallow, it is shallow. Don't try to control the breath. Just let the air out through the nose and back in through the nose again in its natural flow.

As your breathing becomes steady, slowly move your entire attention to a part of your face situated on the entrance of the nostrils, that is above the upper lip bellow the nostrils. Keep your entire attention focused on that area and just observe how the air from the outside is coming in and going out. Coming in and going out. Coming in and going out ...

Why should you concentrate on the breath? With concentrating on your breath you will simply start focusing your mind. The breath is always there, and every human being owns it. This technic probably derives from ancient times, and it is used in many traditions of meditation. It was not me who invented it. I am just using it as a powerful method to calm myself and to focus on important things when there are numerous thoughts wandering through my mind.

As you continue with concentrating and observing the breath as it comes in and goes out, one really interesting thing is going to happen. In just a few moments after you have focused your entire attention to your breath, your mind is probably going to slip somewhere else. It is going to wander away. It could be that you are going to start thinking about breakfast or about some errands or tasks that had to be done that day or you'll be thinking about the words that your spouse told you the other day in anger and you haven't had opportunity to talk them through.

If something like this starts to happen to you, just don't panic. Don't even start to feel angry, disappointed or discouraged. This doesn't mean that you don't know how to meditate or that you did something wrong or that you should quit or anything like that. All these thoughts are perfectly normal. It means that you are doing everything just right. It happens, and it is still happening to everyone who meditates.

What you ought to do is to simply and slowly bring your focused attention back to the area below the nostrils and above the upper lip, and again focus on your breathing however it may be. If your mind is really distracted and you can't bring your focused attention to the area between your nose and mouth then start again from the beginning. Take a few slightly deeper breaths and when your breathing slows down try to focus on the area below the nostrils and above the upper lip again. Do not give too much attention to the content of your thoughts and don't even judge them. Thoughts are just thoughts. They will be there continuously as long as you breathe and live. You can even tell yourself that all these thoughts are perfectly all right, that you accept them as they are. The most important thing is that you don't get too hard on yourself and that you don't judge yourself. Just keep slowly and attentively bringing your attention back to the breath until the alarm clock goes off and the 15 minutes are over.

As you practice focusing on your breathing, try to prolong this exercise for one minute every time you sit. If you meditate once a day, you will be able to prolong it from fifteen minutes to thirty or even forty minutes in twenty days. But if you are really busy and you don't have that time, then you should prolong the exercise each day for two minutes, and in twenty days you should be able to meditate for almost an hour.

My meditation routine now lasts an hour every morning. And I also started with just fifteen minutes each morning for number of days. But in the end, it is really up to you. You are your own master, and you must decide how much of your time you are willing to sacrifice.

Now that you're through your first exercise and your first fifteen minutes, you should congratulate yourself! I congratulate you too! You have just managed to do your first step to a new, better, calmer and more positive YOU. Go on and have a magnificent day.

Chapter 16: Fun activities

You have probably noticed that when you do something you like, your mood improves. If you do something you really enjoy every day your general mood will improve, which is especially important if you are depressed.

Try listing all of the activities you like doing on a piece of paper or on your computer/tablet/cell phone and do at least one activity from the list each day from now on!

When I first wrote my list, I realized that there are so many things I enjoy doing, and it was a huge eye-opening experience for me! I wish you that same feeling!

Make sure that what you do is not hazardous to your health because, if that is the case, it won't help you in the long run, but deteriorate your health.

So for example, if you like drinking hard liquor on your balcony while smoking a cigarette, it's not really helpful in the long run.

But you can smoke an electric cigarette and drink a glass of quality red wine, which contains resveratrol that fights against free radicals in order to prolong your life.

Footnote about resveratrol:

Resveratrol may be the most significant discovery in supplement history. Resveratrol is best known as a red wine molecule, a matchless and distinctive molecule for human health and longevity.

Dr. Sinclair in the famous Harvard study discovered the resveratrol molecule stimulates the SIRT1 gene known as the calorie restriction gene, which is the only gene expression proven to extend human life. In the past ten years, hundreds of studies have been conducted with resveratrol.

It provides a healthy response to so many health concerns including cardiovascular disease, weight loss, cancer, diabetes, cognitive decline, etc. – scientist say its antioxidant benefits alone are miraculous.

Of course, this doesn't mean that you need to drink red wine all the time, but every now and then a glass of quality red wine can be good for you if it doesn't conflict with your medication.

Back to the activities: So it doesn't really matter what activities make you happy, what is important that you do them regularly.

If you like table tennis, you should visit the local sports club and apply for membership. If you like swimming, search for a swimming pool nearby and go there a few times a week.

It could be going to the cinema or the theater or just listening to classical music at home.

By the way, there are some very interesting effects of listening to classical music, after reading about them in the next chapter you might get passionate about them!

Chapter 17: Tricks of the Mind

In case of sudden attacks of anxiety, you might not have the time to reach for a cup of herbal tea, or get out and start running, or even grab a chocolate bar. In cases like this, you can try a few tricks for the purpose of confusing your mind and set it out of its current state.

One such trick is the simplest of them all. Breathe. The concept is that you cannot breathe deeply and be anxious at the same time. A classic yoga trick you can use is the following: Exhale completely from the mouth and then inhale through your nose slowly by counting up to 4 seconds. Hold your breath and count up to 7 seconds. Now exhale slowly through your mouth counting another 8 seconds. Repeat at least twice a day.

Adjusting your mindset will not help only in sudden situations. It is the key to the long term solution to the core fear. Here are a few methods you can try to set your mind to the right path.

When you're attacked by anxiety, it is easy to get into an attitude known as "catastrophizing." Your mind goes to all the bad, terrible, really horrible, just unbearable things and the possibility of them really happening. If and when this occurs, breathe as shown above, take a long walk, and consider the real possibility that any issue will really result to a catastrophe. How probable is it that you will become unemployed, or never talk to your sister again, or go broke? Most of the times we worry about things that are never going to happen. It is important to be able to control our mind and stop it from wandering and worrying about things like these.

A little more advanced practice for the mind is what is called "mindfulness meditation". Initially a Buddhist training, but now a normal treatment, it is particularly effective in treating anxiety. This is achieved by paying attention to the current moment, deliberately, with inquisitiveness, and with an effort to be non-judgmental. How can this be done? This is the real trick. Considering how to do this, will not let you think about your disorder. And when you do figure out how to do this, then you will not be thinking about your anxiety.

Further to the advanced mental functions, another step is to breath and question. To stay mindful by asking yourself simple questions while practicing breathing exercises. To do this, you need to sit comfortably, close your eyes and focus on how your breath feels coming in and out of the body. Then begin asking yourself questions like what is the temperature of the air as it enters your nose, how does the air feel as it fills the lungs, or if it feels differently as it leaves your body. Of course, you are also required to provide the correct answers. This will not only freshen your mind but also help you concentrate on other things instead of issues that are troubling you.

The most valid statement for all kinds of disorders is that, the first step towards a cure is to admit that you have a problem. Therefore, if you recognize at some point that you are having anxious thoughts, you are worthy of congratulations, because you are aware of your emotional state. At this point it is most imperative to give yourself some credit, because this is truly a skill that must be learned, and is essential for the rest of the treating process.

The purpose of all mental exercises is not only to take your mind off the problem. It is also to provide the means to fight the core of your problem through firstly, a better understanding of your own physical and mental condition and secondly, by improving the mental condition which will in turn improve the physical condition.

Chapter 18: Supplements for Depression and Anxiety

It is extremely important for you to consume some supplements when you wish to avail relief from stress and depression. In this chapter we will look at some of the supplements that you need to consume to avail relief from these conditions at the earliest.

Vitamin D

It is believed that a vitamin D deficiency is responsible for the production of cortisol in the brain, which causes stress to increase. So, it might be important for you to get a blood test done and check the level of vitamin D in your body. If there is a deficiency then you should ask your doctor to prescribe the best vitamin D supplement for your body. The dosage will differ from person to person and if you live in an area where there is very little sunlight then you should take a larger dose as compared to those that live in sunny places.

Omega 3 fatty acids

Omega 3 fatty acids are essential for proper brain function. It contains DHA, which is important for brain function and promotes brain health. As per studies conducted on women who suffered from depression, it was found that 30% had this chemical in low levels in their brains. You can consume fish oils for this, as they are extremely rich in omega 3 fatty acids. You can also crush flax seeds and add it to your salads or dissolve in water and consume, as they are extremely rich in omega fatty 3 acids.

Rhodiola

Rhodiola is an herb that is used to treat mental disorders. It is said to help in reducing stress that might be caused due to environmental and physical stimulus. You will feel much calmer and at peace with yourself when you consume this herb and it will also help in reducing your stress and anxiety. Rhodiola is also good with helping in inducing sleep and you will see that most of your worries are starting to shrink. It is available in tablet form and can be bought from online stores.

Gingko

Gingko is an herb that is rich in anti-oxidants and will assist in reducing oxidative damage to the brain. Gingko helps in reducing stress and stress related side effects. It is also used to avail relief from headache and migraine. It helps in increasing the flow of blood to the brain. You will feel much energetic and full of life once you start consuming this herb. It is available in tablet form and can be consumed to avail quick relief from stress.

Lavender

Lavender is an herb that is used in treating stress and anxiety disorders. Lavender is mainly used to induce rest full sleep and will help in reducing your stress and tiredness. You must have used lavender in the form of soaps or shampoos and it is mainly added in for its sweet smell, which is capable of transporting a person to a different world. You can find the fresh stems and flowers of the plant and prepare a calming tea that you can consume to avail relief from your stress and depression. Lavender capsules and oil is also available which you can consume and apply respectively.

Kava kava root

Kava kava is a plant whose root is used to prepare a medicine that is effective in helping people avail relief from stress and anxiety disorders. It is said to be quite potent and has been used since time immemorial to serve this very purpose. Kava kava is also used in treating sleep related disorders such as insomnia and will allow you to avail restful sleep. It is said to help with excess fatigue and will help in reducing the stress that you might have accrued through it.

Passionflower

Passionflower is said to be extremely helpful in providing relief from stress and stress related issues. It helps in reducing anxiety and depression. The flower helps in reducing nervousness and aids in improving confidence. It is also used to treat high blood pressure and will help in keeping you calm and composed. Passionflower is available in the tablet form and can be bought online. It also helps in reducing irregular heartbeats and assists in regularizing the beats.

Valerian root

Valerian root is extremely useful in fighting away disorders of the mind. You can use the herb to avail relief from stress and anxiety related disorders. It has been used in treating asthma that is caused by anxiety and also provides relief from hyperventilation. It is also quite useful in reducing the effects of stress and depression and will aid in increasing the flow of blood to your brain. Valerian root is extremely effective in helping you reduce anxiety and panic attacks. It is available in tablet form and you can but it online.

Gingko

Gingko is an ancient Chinese medicine that is still used to treat memory and mental disorders. Gingko helps in many ways as it affects not just the mind but also the body. Traditionally, the herb was used to aid in relief from Alzheimer's. It is available in powder or tablet form and both can be consumed to avail relief from stress and depression. The leaves are what are used to prepare the medicines that are used to prepare the medicines that are consumed for stress and anxiety. You can buy the tablets online.

St. John's wort

St. John's wort is one of the most common and used herbs for depression and anxiety. It is said to have shown amazing results with those suffering from these mental issues and so, is one of the most prescribed natural supplements. The herb is used to extract oil that is used to administer to these people. Hypercin is the chemical that lies in the root and is said to be effective in reducing the effects of stress on a person's brain. St. John's wort is available as a tablet that can be consumed to avail relief from these conditions.

Ashwagandha

Ashwagandha is a traditional Indian medicine that is used to treat mental disorders. Ashwagandha root and berry is used for this purpose. It is one of the best herbs that you can use to treat your anxiety disorder. It is often compared with Ginseng, which is the Chinese herb used to treat depression and anxiety. You can take this herb in tablet or powder form and avail relief from all your mental ailments. It is also said to be great for children as it helps in improving their memory and concentration. But you have to ask the doctor first before administering it to your child.

It is important for you to ask a doctor about these medicines first as some of them might not suit your body. It is especially important to ask if you are pregnant or are consuming any medicines.

Chapter 19: SECTION TWO

Anxiety

The current medical view

The National Institute of Mental Health (NIMH) in the USA is the largest scientific organisation in the world dedicated to research on mental disorders, including anxiety and depression. The following information comes from this website.

Anxiety is the most common group of mental disorders in America, with an estimated 18 percent of the population effected to some degree. There are many different diagnostic levels of anxiety, some of them being General Anxiety Disorder (GAD), Social Anxiety, Post- traumatic Stress Disorder (PTSD), Obsessive-Compulsive Disorder (OCD) and the various Phobias'.

Panic Disorder

Sudden and repeated attacks of intense fear. Feelings of being out of control during a panic. Intense worries about feeling attacked. Avoidance of places where panic attacks have occurred previously.

Social Anxiety Disorder

Anxious around other people and difficulty in conversation. Feelings of self-consciousness, and worried about feeling humiliated, embarrassed, rejected, fearful of offending others. Afraid of being judged, staying away from people, feeling sick and nauseous in company.

Other Symptoms

Uncontrollable worry, insomnia, obsessive thoughts, muscle tension, feeling on edge, blushing and sweating, rapid heart rate and shortness of breath.

Anxiety creates lack of sleep, an inability to concentrate, irritability, lack of energy and constant worry. These problems can then turn into highly negative thoughts about yourself and may keep you in a worst-case scenario mindset. (from my own personal experience constantly thinking about the worst-case scenario was the main thing I hated about my anxiety. Most of the scenes I imagined happening were gruesomely awful).

There are many websites and personal blogs on the internet that discuss anxiety. Following is a selection of how people experience anxiety.

"When my anxiety is bad I pass out. I throw up, I get dizzy, I lose my vision and hearing and feeling in my body and become numb."

"Imagine waking in the morning and not being able to move any part of your body. Imagine waking up and barely able to breath and feeling like there is a boulder laying on your chest."

"Anxiety for me is a full body response where my body becomes so confused it doesn't know how to respond. I sometimes wonder will I ever be able to survive."

"But one thing remains true for all of us who suffer panic attacks – during them we feel like we will die."

"No matter how calm cool and collected I look, on the inside it's like cats stuck in a storm drain. It is a constant fight to appear normal and is exhausting trying to calm the inner demons."

"I'm frozen with fear, with paranoia, with anxiety. It isn't that I am a man of few words, it's that I'm a brain too many….. and too few all at once."

"Inside, everything is far from calm. I've already run through 160 possible 'what ifs'. Also, don't change the plan – not even a tiny bit, unless you give me lots of advance warning."

Causes and risk factors

Genetic and environmental factors, usually in combination, are the main risk factors (NIMH). Others are shyness in childhood, being female, having few economic resources, divorced or widowed, anxiety in relatives, parental history of mental disorders, elevated afternoon cortisol levels, exposure to stressful life events in childhood and adulthood.

During my early years it was socially acceptable to spank children. Even in the current times there are people who believe that a good spanking did them no harm, and see no reason not to spank their own children. But research is showing how damaging spanking can be. The University of Texas along with the University of Michigan have done 50 years of research on 160,000 children. The short-term results of spanking include antisocial behaviour, depression, increased aggression, misbehaviour and low self-esteem. The long-term effects included antisocial behaviour plus mental illnesses and anxiety later in life.

Research from McGill University has shown that emotional abuse has a similar impact on child development as physical abuse. (these findings fit Primal Theory in the fact it is lack of love that causes mental disorders. Both physical and emotional abuse towards children, or any human for that matter, shows a lack of love. Therefore, the impact on the human brain is the same in both cases.) From my own experience, my father used to belt me occasionally, but the physical side of reliving this trauma did not appear during Primal Therapy. However, the reliving of the emotional abuse and constant fear of living with a 'monster' was a dominate feature. Witnessing the physical violence perpetrated on my younger sisters and my mother caused me a lot of damage. Witnessing of physical violence against another human is one of the things being investigated within the ACE research. The witnessing of physical violence, as opposed to being the victim, seems to be a significant factor of PTSD in war veterans.

Treatments

Anxiety disorders are treated with psychotherapy, medication or both. The NIMH says medication does not cure anxiety but often relieves the symptoms.

Cognitive Behavioural Therapies (CBT) are also common.

Talk therapy - tries to neutralise unhelpful thoughts.

Exposure therapy – confronting your fears

Previously, I mentioned that the three levels of consciousness combined with Primal Theory provide an over-arching paradigm in which to view the human condition. The lack of any solid paradigm shows up in the current medical view on the causes and cures of anxiety, and what is going on in the brain of an anxiety sufferer. There are thousands of books and articles written about anxiety, with dozens of different theories on the causes and many more approaches to treatment. Despite this plethora of information, I have found many blogs where people are spending a lifetime battling the horror and life-limiting effects of severe anxiety and panic attacks.

Following are some of the more common views on how to deal with anxiety.

Three Mindfulness tips to Reduce Anxiety, by Narine Vander Hooven LCSW.

Regulate your breathing - when you are focusing in the moment on your breath, and only on your breath, it's hard to focus on anything else.

Use your senses - focus on seeing, touch, hearing, smell, taste.

Engage in an activity – like colouring books for that purpose or play a musical instrument.

Another headline reads – "Six Ways to Stop Worrying About Things You Can't Control."

'There is a brutal truth in life that some people refuse to accept. You have no control over many of the things that happen in your life. Some people who resist this truth become control freaks. They micromanage, refuse to delegate tasks and try to force other people to change. They think that if they can gain enough control over other people and the situation they find themselves in they can prevent bad things from happening.'

Determine what you can control

Focus on your influence

Identify your fears

Differentiate between ruminating and problem solving

Create a plan to manage your stress

Develop healthy affirmations.

Another viewpoint and advice on how to deal with a particular problem.

The headline - "How to Help Clients Reclaim what has been Lost in Trauma."

'In the moment of trauma, both brain and body quickly adapt to help us survive the event. But later these adaptations can sometimes do more harm than good. For instance, the nervous system may get stuck and shut down or go into overdrive without a client's awareness or conscious choice. To help clients take back control of their brain and body, we've got to be able to teach them how to calm the nervous system. In this short course, Ruth Lanius M.D. PhD, will give you specific interventions to help your client recover what has been lost.' **(The interventions suggested by Lanius were typically intellectually based, with no reference for the need to fix the problem in the basement).**

F.E.A.R. False Evidence Appearing Real is another way of looking at fear. In the case of F.E.A.R., the therapist tries to reason with the sufferer that the situation is not as bad as it seems. This is another theory from the orthodoxy that aggravates me because of my personal experience. The sufferer is feeling some anxiety about the present moment, which resonates at the lower level of brain functioning, where the original threat was very real, and maybe even life-threatening. I regarded myself as having low grade anxiety, but when I entered the basement of my mind during therapy, the terror I experienced was overwhelming and took many sessions to deal with. The original situation was a whole lot worse than I could have imagined. (During JPT the therapist would never invalidate any feelings by saying they may not be real. We validate all feelings and understand that most of them are just the tip of the feeling iceberg.)

The current state of the medical industry is that they are still theorising on the causes of anxiety, attempting to deal with the multitude of symptoms, and applying what I would describe as a haphazard and multi-modal approach to treatment and attempted cure. Compare this situation to the next few pages where I will explain how anxiety has only one main cause, extravagant diagnostics are not needed for treatment, and there is only one path to cure (as opposed to control or management of symptoms).

Chapter 20: NLP Hacks To Replace Anxiety With Happiness

NLP stands for Neuro-linguistic programming, an approach to improving yourself through changing your communication and working on self-development. There exists scores of NLP techniques that can help you become a better, more confident, happier and successful person.

Below are some foolproof NLP techniques you can use to feel happy instantly and curb your anxiety.

1: Anchor Happiness to Your Mind

Anchoring is one of the most effective NLP techniques; it helps you anchor a certain response or emotion to a gesture so that each time you practice that gesture, you enjoy that response. To feel instantly happy, anchor happiness to a hand gesture and imbed it in your subconscious.

Think of a time in your life when you felt extremely happy and concentrate on that experience. Build up to the point when you felt the happiest and enjoy that feeling. Now use a hand gesture to anchor that happiness to it. You could snap your fingers or press two fingers together. Do this a few times while thinking of that happy memory.

Now think of something else and practice that hand gesture. If you have successfully anchored happiness to it, you will instantly recall that memory and feel good. If not, try it a few more times and until you successfully anchor happiness to a hand gesture.

2: Try the Halo Technique

The halo technique boosts your mood within minutes. Think of yourself as protected by a beautiful, bright halo of goodness that keeps every ounce of negativity away from you and makes you feel happy and confident at all times.

Imagine that halo growing bigger, brighter, and stronger as you think more about it. Think of all the good things you can and imagine them being a part of that halo. Smile as you think of these things. You will start feeling better. Put this halo on your head and around yourself every time you feel upset and anxious; whenever you do, you will smile instantly.

3: Circle of Excellence

Similar to the halo technique, this NLP hack makes you feel good about yourself; it helps you forget your worries instantly. Imagine a big circle in front of you and fill it with all the good virtues you can think of such as peace, happiness, sincerity, honesty, confidence, etc.

Now imagine stepping into that circle and absorbing all its goodness. Every nice thing in the circle is entering your body and is now becoming a part of you. For instance, if you were anxious and unhappy with yourself, you are now peaceful and extremely delighted with yourself.

After being in it for some time, step outside the circle and imagine it growing smaller. When it becomes tiny, pick it up, put it in your pocket or wallet, and then take it out whenever anxiety attacks you. You will be up and smiling in no time.

Use these tactics and you will be amazed at what it can do for you:

CHAPTER 21: IMPROVE YOUR CONCENTRATION

Focus takes a great deal of commitment. Even though you practice it for just one week or perhaps a month, the result will not be effective if the human brain isn't carrying out well. Still, there are simple enough ways to boost your focus quickly and effectively.

Long-Term Solutions

Take rest. The largest factor affecting focus is rest which has been approved by research. Focus requires your brain to be relaxed. However your brain will be spread if you aren't well rested. Ensure that you get the right amount of rest at the right time. Likewise have regular rest time, which is the main element step for focusing.

Sleeping too much is not ideal also. Oversleeping disrupts your natural tempo and can cause you to lazy. Avoid this having noisy alarms to wake you up with time.

Make an idea. Always have an idea for whatever you are up to. When you sit back to work without a plan, you might easily get captured in pursuits like looking at mails, instant messaging (chatting) and browsing the net. Without a purpose, you are losing your time and effort. You'll end up distracted by a number of nagging thoughts rather than devoting all of your focus on one important job.

In order to avoid this, make a definite plan that fulfills your requirements beforehand. Take 5 or ten minutes break among, and utilize this time to check on email, and then close your inbox and get to your most significant job. When making an idea make sure to allocate plenty of time for entertainment, studies and rest.

The practice of meditation will improve our powers of concentration definitely. Actually, whenever we make an effort to meditate, it is focus that is the very first thing we have to master. A regular period of meditation gives us the opportunity to work specifically on focus techniques.

Choose a host to your decision for focus. Certainly some places are much better than others. School libraries, research lounges and private rooms will be the best. Most importantly, the area that you select shouldn't be distracting. Try to avoid other people if you would like to focus on your work.

If you wish to grasp the arts of focus, develop a managed and balanced diet. Overeating creates an enormous weight of digestive function and can cause you to feel uncomfortable and sleepy. Eating light and healthy foods will help you increase your capability to focus. As Thomas Jefferson said, we hardly ever regret eating inadequate. It's likely you'll find that you'll require less food to fulfill yourself than you think.

Exercise frequently. The capability to concentrate is dependent a great deal upon our physical well-being. If we are exhausted, harmful and suffering from numerous small illnesses, focus could be more difficult. Of course, concentration is possible still, but it is merely more difficult. However, we must make an effort to make life possible for ourselves; we have to provide a high priority to your physical health:

Getting sufficient sleep

Staying fit physically

Keeping healthy weight

Getting regular physical exercise

Take breaks and blend up your environment. Constant work in the same place can drive anyone crazy. Taking continuous breaks can solve the problem. This can make you energetic and more thinking about your topic.

Understand that practice makes perfect. Focus can be an activity like any other. Obviously the greater we practice, the better our focus can be. We wouldn't be prepared to be considered a strong runner without doing some training. Likewise, concentration is similar to a muscle, the greater we exercise the more powerful it becomes.

Quick Fixes

Make a tally of each time your mind wanders on a 3x5 card. Divide the cards up into three areas: morning, night and afternoon. Each and every time you capture your brain wandering, make just a little checkmark in the correct box. After a little while, viewers your brain won't wander normally, by just keeping a tally!

Being conscious of the problem is the first rung on the ladder, which method can help you stay very alert to every time you lose your focus. Your knowing of what you're doing will eventually help you improve your focus, with no added effort.

With this technique, you'll eventually have the ability to identify your most susceptible times. Say you find a great deal of tallies through the morning hours, if you are still tired as well as your mind will probably drift. That is clearly an indication that you ought to be improving your focus by getting ultimately more rest, or eating a wholesome breakfast.

Reserve specific times throughout the day to be able to let your brain wander or your focus drift. When you have an arranged time throughout the day - say your "drift off" time reaches 5:30 every day, when you reunite from college or work - you might be less inclined to sanction drifting off during 11 a.m. or 3 p.m. In the event that you capture yourself drifting off during the unsanctioned times, inform yourself you have a specified drift off time and make an effort to keep the human brain focused on whatever job is at hands.

Help enhance the circulation of air to the mind. Blood is the primary vehicle of air in our body. But blood gets pooled in the lower half of our bodies consequently of gravity, and doesn't drive as much air to the mind, where it can help improve concentration. To be able to help oxygenate the mind, get right up and go for a walk once in awhile to get the bloodstream pumping.

If you're trapped at work and also you can't really carve out enough time for exercise, try exercising at the office. These range from a variety of things, including isometric or cardio exercises.

Be sure you give the human brain an instant break at least every hour, for the most part every thirty minutes. If your brain has to concentrate regularly for hours at a time, it loses control power as well as your focus levels slip. Easier to space assembling your project out and take breaks or power naps among to be able to reboot your focus and keep it humming at nearer to 100%.

Practice doing a very important factor at the same time, and carrying it out to completion. If you jump everywhere and start a fresh task before you've completed the last one, you're informing your brain that it is okay to change from one at the mercy of another. In the event that you actually want to improve your focus, you'll start wanting to convince the human brain to complete one job before you move onto another one.

Apply this viewpoint to as much different jobs in your daily life as possible. It may seem that completing one book prior to starting the other has nothing in connection with finishing focus on one car prior to starting focus on another, but they're remarkably alike if you believe about. Even the tiniest duties have reverberations in other areas you will ever have.

Be familiar with the spider technique. What goes on when you possess a vibrating tuning fork next to an online with a spider in it? The spider involves investigate where in fact the sound is via since it pays to be interested. But what goes on if you frequently keep a vibrating tuning fork next to the spider's lair? After some time, the spider won't stop to research the tuning fork any longer. It knows what things to expect, so that it ignores it.

The spider technique is behaving similar to the spider. Expect for interruptions to come and make an effort to toss you off your focus. A hinged door slams. A bird whistles. A flash mob erupts. Regardless of the distraction is, continue concentrating on your job at hand. End up like the spider and change a blind vision to distractions you know can toss you off your focus.

Do just work at a table, not your bed. Your bed is where you rest; your table is where you work and focus. Your brain makes these types or associations subconsciously, meaning you're sending a "rest" transmission to your brain if you're seeking to focus on your bed. That is counterproductive because you're actually requesting the human brain to do a couple of things simultaneously (focus and rest). Instead, ask you brain to either focus or rest by choosing your workstation carefully.

Try the five-more guideline. The five-more guideline is simple. Whenever you feel just like giving up or dropping focus, tell you to ultimately do five more of whatever you were doing. Whether it's mathematics problems, do five more problems. Whether it's reading, do five more WebPages. If it's focusing, do five more minutes. Find the power deep within to do five more of whatever you were you doing.

Keywords Technique

Try the Keywords Technique. With this simple technique, the thing you should do is to get the right keyword on what you are learning or doing and once you lose focus or feel sidetracked or your brain wanders to another thing, start that keyword frequently in your thoughts until you get back to the topic accessible. The keyword in this system is not really a single, set term but maintains changing relating to your research or work. You will find no rules to choose the keyword and whichever phrase the individual feels that it'll recreate his focus can be utilized as a keyword.

Example: If you are reading articles about your guitar. Here the keyword acoustic guitar can be utilized. Start reading each phrase gradually even though reading, once you feel sidetracked or unable to understand or focus, start stating the keyword electric guitar, acoustic guitar, electric guitar, acoustic guitar, guitar until your mind comes back to the article and you can continue your reading then. And make a habit to do meditation for at least ten minutes which enhances your focus levels. Nevertheless, you see that you merely focus on deep breathing first for better improvement or effect.

Chapter 22: The power of positive thinking

The thoughts that often play in our head and oftentimes replay over and over, directly control how we feel. The good news? You may not have complete control of every single. That pops in your mind, but you do have control over what you choose to focus on!

Anytime you hear that negative thought, or compulsive back, hit that delete button, or rejection button inside of your mind. Don't dwell on that thought. What you focus on will get bigger and grow. Whether that's negative negative or positive.

Think of your mind sort of like a magnifying glass. Whatever the magnifying glass focuses on, it gets bigger right? Or the same applies to your mind. Whatever you focus on will be bigger and stronger

So all that time that you spend focused on how to feel better, how to treat anxiety, how to feel normal again. That's just magnifying your situation and making your anxiety more intense. Again it's a cycle

Chapter 23: Mindfulness Meditation

Mindfulness meditation can clear your mind, positively shift your emotional state, help manage stress, and reduce anxiety. It simply involves directing your focus and attention to the present moment, without judging or analyzing the present as good or bad, happy or sad. It encourages living in the moment – even a painful or sad moment – as fully and as mindfully as possible. Mindfulness is more than a relaxation technique; it's an attitude towards stress and anxiety. With mindfulness, you focus your mind on the present moment, without any intention of improving or changing anything. Observing and accepting life as it is, with all its disappointments, pains, frustrations, insecurities, joys, and pleasures, enables you to become more confident, calm, and able to cope with whatever happens.

Sit comfortably in a chair or on the floor with your head, neck, and back straight. Try these steps:

Focus on a single thing, such as your breathing. Concentrate on the feeling of the air as it enters and exits with each breath. Don't try to control your breathing too much by slowing it down or speeding it up; just observe as it is.

Even when you are determined to focus on your breathing, your mind will wander. When this happens, notice where your mind went; perhaps you drifted to your work schedule or a negative past experience. Observe, and then gently return your attention to your breathing.

Use your breathing as an anchor. Every time a distracting feeling or thought arises, briefly acknowledge it. Don't judge it or analyze it; just observe it, and then return to your breathing.

Let go of all thoughts of future events, wishes, duties, and plans. Keep threading moments of mindfulness together, breath by breath.

Start with 5 minutes of practice, or even just a minute at a time. You can gradually increase the time to 10, 20, or even 30 minutes as your focus improves over time.

Chapter 24: Recovering and Rediscovering

We have begun the initial stage of your recovery through your acceptance and commitment, and have set up the framework for your journey with the 30 day rejection therapy challenge, but it is now time to delve into the main body of work. These are steps to be taken during the 30 day challenge, they compliment it and enhance it, and, will in turn be complimented and enhanced by it.

You can choose your own schedule to follow, but you must have completed all of the steps by the time the 30 days are up if you want to see some real progress. It will be hard and intimidating, you will be pushed far out of your comfort zone and awaken emotions and memories that you have suppressed, but this is all for your own good. Whenever you feel like giving up and letting your social anxiety control you, remember the commitment you made, and remember why you made it.

The Five Pillars of Treatment

There are five main stations on the journey through your treatment:

1) Redirecting Your Thinking

2) Learning to Control Your Breath

3) Facing Your Fears

4) Building Better Relationships

5) Changing Your Lifestyle

They are the pillars of your recovery, and should be moved through in step.

1) Redirecting Your Thinking

Negative thoughts that stem from and, in turn, fueling a distorted world view are one of the fundamental contributors to social anxiety disorder. If you are suffering, you will undoubtedly be familiar with intrusive and destructive thoughts like "**I know I'm going to embarrass myself**", "**My voice, hands, feet or body is going to fail me know**", "**I'm not cool or interesting enough to be here**" etc...

In order to combat the disorder, you need to start challenging these thoughts. This can be done with the help of a therapist, but it can also be done by yourself.

The first step is to recognize irrational, negative thoughts when you have them. For example, when you have a presentation coming and think "**I'm not good enough to do this, I'm going to blow it**". Once you flag these thoughts, think about them and challenge them. In this case, you clearly are good enough to give the presentation or you wouldn't be in the position, and, even if you are nervous when you speak, that doesn't mean that people will see you as incompetent.

Once you have begun to challenge these basic negative thoughts, you can then work on redirecting your thinking. At first this will be challenging, but with practice it will begin to feel natural. People with social anxiety disorder often waste time on the following follies:

Mind Reading: Assuming that you know what others are thinking, and specifically, assuming that they are thinking negative thoughts about you. No disrespect, but they probably have other things on their minds.

Predicting the (Negative) Future: Assuming that things will go horribly wrong before they even happen. This will make you anxious about situations before they begin.

Dramatization: Blowing things out of proportion, i.e thinking that if you wear the wrong thing to school everybody will judge you and your life will be ruined forever. It won't. People won't care, and if they do, they will have forgotten by the next day.

Personalization: Assuming that other people's reactions relate to you in some way. For example, thinking that someone isn't going to a party just because you are attending. Again, no disrespect, but you're probably not that big of a concern to them.

Once you are aware of these thought patterns, you can acknowledge them and put a stop to them. Do not let yourself indulge such fantasies, they are simultaneously narcissistic and inhibiting, and that is not a good combination.

Just being aware of these pitfalls isn't always enough to overcome them of course, so here is some proven advice for getting over the feeling that everyone is watching you:

• Reduce your self focus by giving attention instead to things that are going on around you; look at other people and the surroundings rather than thinking about your own actions and bodily symptoms of anxiety.

• Don't always feel the need to make conversation. Not all silence is awkward, and if you take a minute, someone else will say something.

- Really listen to what is happening around you (either conversation wise or background noise like the radio) instead of focusing on your negative thoughts.

2) Controlling Your Breathing

When you start to feel anxious, your body is overwhelmed by a number of physical symptoms which then make you panic even more. One of the most universal of these is an increase in the speed that you breathe. Breathing too fast throws off the balance of oxygen and carbon dioxide in your body, and this gives rise to other symptoms of anxiety such as dizziness, fast and heavily pounding heart beat, and muscle and facial tension.

Practice the following breathing exercise to lower your breathing speed and stay calm in stressful social situations:

-Sit/stand comfortably with your shoulders relaxed and your back straight.

-Inhale slowly through your nose for four seconds.

-Hold the breath in for two seconds.

- Exhale slowly from your mouth for six seconds, pushing out as much air as possible.

-Continue this steady pattern and focus on it.

3) Facing Your Fears

You will already be doing this on a daily basis with the rejection therapy challenge, but the next step is to overcome your fear of specific social situations. To do this, you need to face the kind of events you would normally avoid head on. Treat them as a challenge to be conquered, and understand that it is your avoidance that perpetuates your social anxiety. Once you embrace these situations, the fear will lose all of its power over you.

Avoidance will also prevent you from reaching your goals and achieving what you are truly capable of. Think about it, you could be an amazing song writer and musician, but unless you show people your ideas, no one will ever appreciate it.

Again, like rejection therapy, this is to be approached in stages. Don't tackle your fears straight away, but work up to them in steps. For example, if you are afraid of meeting new people, go with a friend to a party, or even just spend your lunch break with them in the company of others. When you get comfortable with this, then you can try to talk with the other people in similar situations more directly, and eventually, you will be able to go to places by yourself and have conversations with people you have never met before.

Also, use the skills you have learned in other steps to control your breathing, challenge your negative thoughts and stay calm.

4) Build Better Relationships

Actively engaging in encouraging social environments is another excellent way of conquering social anxiety disorder. By finding inviting and non-intimidating social activities to take part in, you will be able to interact with people without putting yourself under extreme amounts of pressure.

Some examples of these include:

• **Social Skills/Assertive Training Classes:** These are offered in many local schools and colleges as night courses. Not only will they help you to improve your confidence and social skills, they will allow you to mix with people who are struggling in the same way as you, and thus, provide you with an excellent support network.

• **Volunteer Work in Something You Enjoy:** It could be helping out in an animal shelter or putting up posters for a band, what matters is getting out and doing something in an area that interests you while getting to meet like-minded people.

• **Taking Hobby Classes:** If you like to draw, take up an art class. If you like reading, join a book club or even a creative writing class. Again, the goal here is to stimulate and develop your interests in the company of people who are doing the same thing.

5) Change Your Lifestyle

A healthier lifestyle can seriously help your recovery. Your body is fueled by food and maintained by sleep and exercise, so it is little wonder that these elements have a huge impact on how it functions. Make positive changes, and you will soon experience the benefits.

- **Limit Your Caffeine Intake:** Caffeine stimulates your body by sending it in to a state of panic, and unsurprisingly this increases the symptoms of anxiety. Tea, coffee, energy drinks, soda and even some chocolate bars contain high amounts of caffeine and should be avoided as much as possible.

- **Rethink Your Drinking:** In the short term drinking can seem like a way of calming your nerves in social events, but in the long run it can lead to an abundance of mental health issues and increase your levels of anxiety. Even people without social anxiety often report suffering from "The Fear" after a night of heavy drinking!

- **Stop Smoking:** Nicotine is a powerful stimulant, and, despite common misconceptions, after the immediate act or smoking, your anxiety levels will have risen, not lowered.

- **Get Enough Sleep:** Sleeping repairs your brain, and you should get 8 hours a night. If you do not get enough sleep you will be far more vulnerable to anxiety. As the old saying goes "**Tiredness makes cowards of us all**".

- **Get Some Exercise:** Do not underestimate the importance of regular exercise. Even 30 minutes a day will transform your well being, and a healthy body really does lead to a healthy mind. Also, exercise has the additional benefit of releasing endorphins, these are chemicals in your brain that make you feel happy and relaxed.

Acknowledging and Confronting Your Fears

We have talked about the importance of facing your fears as one of the five pillars of your treatment, and you should be doing this in some way everyday as part of rejection therapy, so you are probably wondering why we are devoting another section to it?

Well, the reason is this: Your disorder is one that centers almost entirely around irrational fear. It may sound harsh and demanding, but the crux of your recovery is based on confronting and overcoming that fear. Any therapist will tell you the same, except they will charge you a lot more!

You need to acknowledge, understand and conquer the things that spark your anxiety. So, without delay, right now, without reading any further, you need to make a list of ten social situations that you are afraid of. Get a pen and paper and start writing. Do not be apprehensive, this is an extremely exciting moment. You are getting ready for a battle, initiating change, and about to regain control of your life.

If you are having trouble focusing at first, take a look at the following suggestions, but make sure to personalize them and add your own.

- Meeting new people
- Being the center of attention
- Being watched while doing work
- Engaging in small talk
- Public speaking
- Performing on stage
- Being teased or criticized
- Talking with "important"/"cool" people or authority figures
- Being asked a question in class
- Going on a date
- Talking on the phone
- Using public bathrooms
- Taking exams
- Eating or drinking in public
- Speaking up in a meeting

- Going to parties or other social events

You should be proud of yourself for taking immediate action and creating your list, it shows determination and dedication, but the work doesn't simply stop there. That's okay though, nothing worth having comes easy.

You now need to to take your list and, at the end of each situation write a score. This score is from a scale of 1-10, regarding how frightening each activity seems to you, with 10 being terrifying and un-achievable, and 1 being something you could do right now without any problems (there shouldn't be any 1's on your score card... yet).

Next, as your confidence improves and you face your fears bit by bit, in the way outlined above, you need to document each stage. For example, if you are terrified of performing on stage or in front of a crowd, but you like to play music, start by playing to a friend. Casually play something and ask what they think. Before doing so, write down how scared the thought made you feel, and then after you have done it, write down another score correlating to how scary it seems to you now. The second score will be much lower. Continue this as you face your fear in steps, for example, you might next play in front of your family, then you can try to play with a band... and eventually you will be able to get up on stage and play.

Keep these lists, they are the markers of your recovery. Constantly push your boundaries, and as you see how the before score is much higher than the after score, you will not only realize that irrational fear is at the root of your problem, you will defeat it.

And, finally, when you have faced your fears, rewrite a new overall score beside the initial one. It will be much lower, because you will be much more confident.

Chapter 25: Body Scan Meditation- Why Do it and How to Do it

Body scan meditation a powerful meditative technique that helps you relax your body and eliminate the stress accumulated in it. With this meditation technique, all you have to do is to gently and non-judgmentally observe and scan your body parts, one by one while lying down comfortably. Mostly, it begins with observing your toes and ends up with scanning your head.

Why Practice Body Scan Meditation

Stress does not only affect your mind but also your body. When routine stress is not managed on time, it manifests itself in the shape of headaches, body aches, backaches and different kinds of bodily tensions. By practicing body scan meditation, you can get rid of all that unattended stress in your body. As you do away with the stress affecting your body parts, your body feels lighter, calmer and healthier.

Moreover, eliminating stress from your body also helps you become more focused and grounded. When there is nothing distracting you, you can focus easily on the task at hand.

In addition, body scan meditation is a great technique, which you can use to become more accepting of your body. Often, we are not pleased with our bodies or a certain part of our body and don't feel good about it. For instance, if you have a bulging belly, you may not like yourself because of it and may develop a negative attitude because of it. This unaccepting attitude towards yourself makes you nurture self-hate, which does nothing but sabotage your well-being. You can turn this self-hate into self-acceptance and self-love by observing your body nonjudgmentally and becoming more accepting of it. Body scan meditation teaches you to accept yourself as you are without nurturing any negativity for it. If you feel unhappy with something, you need to figure out how to improve it and not just think badly about it. Therefore, if you don't like that you are obese, work towards getting a slimmer body but hating your body will not help you in any way. When you nurture a positive, nonjudgmental attitude towards your body, you start loving it, which consequently encourages you to take healthier decisions for yourself.

Now that you are aware of the many reasons why body scan meditation should be a part of your routine, let us find out how to do it.

How to Practice Body Scan Meditation

Usually, a body scan meditation session lasts from anywhere between 20 to 60 minutes but if you are pressed for time, you can do it for 10 to 15 minutes as well. Here's what you need to do to practice this powerful meditation technique.

1: Lie Down Comfortably

Choose a quiet, peaceful room to meditate in. Lie down comfortably on the floor or on a yoga mat or even on the bed if the floor is too hard and uncomfortable for you. Make sure to lie straight on your back and spread your legs about 2 inches apart from each other. Keep your arms to your sides but not too close to the body. Your palms should face upwards. You can keep your eyes closed or open as you please.

2: Register Your Attitude

Once you are lying comfortably, become conscious of the attitude you are nurturing right now. Whatever it is that you are feeling, register and acknowledge it. If you are angry, happy, sad, depressed or calm- acknowledge those feelings without attaching any labels or extra emotions to them. Make sure not to tell yourself to improve your anger issues or let go of your stress and avoid advising anything to yourself.

Mindfulness is about allowing yourself to feel what you are feeling without being judgmental of it so let your emotions flow and accept them.

3: Bring Your Attention to Your Breath

Gently bring your attention to your breath and observe it for a few minutes. Stay with your breath for a few moments and you will find yourself feeling more grounded. Breathe in your natural manner and don't deepen or lengthen your breath.

4: Start Observing Your Body

After a few minutes of observing your breath, bring your attention to your toes and observe them very closely. Focus on the sensations you are feeling; any pain in your toes or any sort of strain you experience. If you nurture any sort of judgment or negative feeling about your toes, acknowledge it and then let go of it. Think of how helpful your toes are and all the reasons why you should be thankful for them and you'll start feeling happier about them. Scan your toes for a few minutes and you'll feel a lot relaxed than before.

Gradually, move to your feet, legs, torso, chest and so on till you get to the top of your head. Analyze each part the same way, letting go of any judgement or label attached to it as you scan it. Be very gentle and accepting with each body part and observe it patiently.

After you have scanned all your body parts, imagine that your breath is a wave of fresh air and is sweeping all the way up and down your entire body. It begins entering your toes and reaches the top of the head in one swift, smooth motion. As your breath moves through your body, it brings in peace and removes any stress in it.

When you feel relaxed or when you feel it is time for you to end the practice, gradually bring your awareness to the world around you. Stop analyzing your body and imagining your breath sweeping up and down the body and just relax. When your awareness returns to the real world, slowly get up. Make sure to record all your observations in a journal to track your performance. Moreover, it also helps you understand why you aren't accepting of your body and how you can improve. In addition, it helps you figure out the areas most affected by stress and how body scan meditation helps relieve that stress.

Practice it daily and soon, you'll start loving yourself even more.

Chapter 26: Internal Stressors

Anxiety and panic are caused by our reaction to things inside us as well as to things outside us. In short, we often create our own anxiety problems by escalating insignificant experiences to full-blown panic attacks. Here's how we do this to ourselves:

Random physical sensations.

The body is continually interacting with and adapting to the environment. We experience this exchange in innumerable ways, a few of which are listed here:

changes in body temperature and breathing pattern

sensitivity to light and noise

internal twinges and muscle twitching

stomach rumblings and pain, nausea

tight chest, jaw, minor aches and pains

quickly shifting emotions, irritability

Most people accept these changing physical sensations as normal. But others who are afraid of having anxiety symptoms and panic attacks, or have PTSD, tend to overreact and in doing so escalate normal body sensations into more intense physical, anxiety symptoms and emotions.

Low-level anxiety symptoms.

Low-level anxiety symptoms can and often do trigger more intense anxiety symptoms. People who fear having panic attacks often overreact to minor anxiety symptoms that when overlooked often go away. When low-level anxiety symptoms are noticed quietly without reacting, they often disappear on their own. But when minor symptoms are perceived as dangerous, a panic-feedback loop is set in motion. Unless anxiety-management strategies are used at this point, minor symptoms can escalate to full-blown panic.

Catastrophic thinking.

Imagining the worst-case scenario, dwelling on it, and creating an anxious state is the hallmark of all anxiety disorders. When anyone has thoughts that begin with **"What if"** and envision horrible things happening in the future—without seeking a solution— it is called catastrophic thinking. Fear-based thoughts are more than mental constructs; they are also chemical messengers that activate the **fight-flight-freeze** nervous system and are capable of escalating anxiety to panic.

Catastrophic thoughts are capable of causing panic attacks, because the **fight-flight-freeze** response does not differentiate between real or perceived threats. Geared to err on the side of caution in case the threat is real, the body prepares to protect itself by becoming physically aroused every time it feels threatened.

For example, a person with a flying phobia could trigger the **fight-flight-freeze** response simply by imagining himself on an airplane, and the physiological arousal would be the same as if he were actually on the airplane.

The **good news** is that you can use your imagination to change how you feel for the better and to improve your performance in all things. Because positive visualization has been shown to improve athlete's performance more than physical practice does, it is widely used in professional sports as a winning strategy.

Anna had a driving phobia that began when she got in the car. From the passenger seat, I saw worry cross her face the moment the garage door opened and worsen when she started the engine. In several seconds, Anna had escalated to full blown panic. 'What are you thinking?' I asked. In an outpouring of fear, she cried, "I'm afraid my foot will accidentally hit the gas, shoot the car out into traffic, crash, and you will be killed." I realized right then how much our thoughts determine behavior. I had Anna turn off the engine and together we brought her anxiety level down. When she was calmer, we visualized a new scenario with a successful outcome. After that, Anna was calm enough to keep her thoughts positive, her arousal under control, and to continue practicing driving.

Unexpressed emotions.

Not being honest about our feelings—not expressing deeply held emotions—is a common cause of anxiety and panic. Remember, the body is always on our side trying to insure our safety and wellbeing. When you hide something that is really important to you, you create an inner disturbance that is often expressed as anxiety.

Anxiety is a shill for other emotions.

Emotions such as anger, rage, unhappiness, guilt, embarrassment, and shame can be scary to express and painful to hear, therefore they can be difficult to express. For some people, it may be safer to have anxiety problems than it is to be honest about how they feel, especially in challenging situations where loss and reprisal are possible consequences.

It is well known that people with anxiety issues are **people pleasers** who sacrifice what they value to keep others happy. Although this strategy may avoid conflict for a short while, it is ineffective and unhealthy for everyone in the long run.

Although the person hiding his or her emotions may not be conscious of doing so, the body keeps the score and expresses them as anxiety, seemingly random physical sensations, illness, and/or accidents.

The way inhibited emotions are communicated and expressed as physical sensations and symptoms (such as anxiety and panic attacks) is called somatization.

The information in the table below is drawn from my observations of clients over the years and from Heal Your Body by Louise Hay.

Table 1

Emotions	Somatic Expression of Repressed Emotion
Pleasure & Joy	Low grade stomach/head aches, muscle tension, bitterness, viral infections, boredom, restlessness, resentment, heaviness, depression, unhappiness, discontented
Anger	Tight jaw, grinding teeth, tight neck/shoulders, fever, depression, closed fist, chronic fatigue, revenge, passive aggression, irritability, arthritis, IBS, tachycardia, autonomic arousal, rash behavior, eye

	problems, kidney stones, lupus, sties, sore throat, warts, blushing, red-faced, dyspareunia
Love	Eating disorders, heart pain/problems, bitterness, low self-esteem, craving sweets, heaviness, cold feet, nose bleeds, numbness
Grief	Tight chest, lump in throat, clogged sinuses, invisible tears, emotional numbness, lung problems, hyperventilation, sadness, crying, isolation, housebound, loneliness
Affection	Psoriasis, aches, rashes, blushing, shyness, dislikes being touched
Sex	Back pain, irritability, horny, dry itchy skin, tenseness, eating disorders, psychosomatic aches/pains, middle finger pain, vaginitis, migraines, urinary

	infections, vaginismus
Hurt	Anger, withdrawn, emotionally isolated, depression, tender to the touch
Wanting	Anger, envy, hopelessness, despair, jealousy, bitterness, victimhood
Guilt	Addictions, apathy, back problems, impotence, pain, shame
Fear	Hyperventilation, frigidity, lump in throat, nervousness, anxiety symptoms, gas pains, hives, nausea, hyperactivity, indigestion, insomnia, overweight, paralysis, ulcers, shingles, tics, phobias

CHAPTER 27: MEDITATE FOR PERSONAL DISCOVERY

Meditation is a practice of mindfulness and focus that makes it possible for you to get important insights about yourself and the world around you. For all those seeking to better understand themselves and experience self-discovery, meditation will help you quiet your brain and better evaluate your daily life. However, deep breathing alone won't give you personal insights. By regularly meditating and living a far more thoughtful life, you might be in a position to better understand who you are and what you can handle.

Practicing Meditation

Find a calm place. Before you start meditating, you should find a silent place that is free from any interruptions. Ensure that there is certainly nothing at all in the area that may break your focus. Switch off all gadgets or leave them in another room. Stay away from places with plenty of individuals or which have heavy feet traffic. When there is outside sound that you find distracting, consider playing some smooth ambient music.

Get comfortable. To be able to facilitate your meditation, you should get as comfortable as possible. You should wear lose fitted clothes that inhale easily. Make sure to take a seat on or cushioning in a manner that is comfortable for you. Although professionals of deep breathing tend to be depicted seated cross-legged, this isn't an essential present. However, you should sit down in a way that facilitates your deep breathing, so make sure to keep the back straight.

If you plan to make meditation a normal practice, you might consider investing in a meditation cushion. You may be thinking about walking meditation. However, this is normally done by more complex professionals. Avoid prone, which might make you drift off. With deep breathing, you desire to be relaxed yet notify.

State your targets. When you are in an appropriate position, condition to yourself what you would like out of your practice. If you're looking for self-discovery, say things such as "I wish to know myself better" or "find my advantages." Saying your targets gives your practice purpose and help you better concentrate. Make an effort to make your goal a mantra. For instance, "power" or "knowledge" may be good mantras for self-discovery.

Close your eye. After you condition your targets, close your eye. In your thoughts, check out how the body feels. Focus on and investigate any feelings which come along. Take the time and psychologically undertake your body, analyzing all its feelings.

Emphasize your respiration. Take deep breaths in and out. You should fill up your lungs with air and gradually release it. Focus on your deep breathing and the motion of the body.

Try to inhale and exhale from your diaphragm. This can help you ingest more air and sluggish your breathing, assisting you relax.

Concentrate. Once you've started your respiration, continue to focus on each breathing. Place all your attention on your inhaling and exhaling. This frees your brain from the strain and stress that can cloud it.

You might like to try duplicating a mantra to help you concentrate. That is a term that you'll do it again to help your concentrate and express your purpose. For instance, if you want to better understand yourself, try mantras like "truth," "finding" or "genuine."

You may even find that taking a look at a graphic or fixed object helps your practice. Some individuals focus by looking at the fire of the candle.

Enhancing Your Meditation Practice

Meditate consistently. To be able to strengthen your practice and keep on your trip of self-discovery, you'll need to meditate regularly. For introspective meditation, you should practice for 10-20 minutes every day or for at least three to four 4 days weekly. This regular practice alters the human brain activity by conditioning the elements of your brain linked to empathy and understanding yourself as well as others.

The take action of disciplining and committing you to ultimately a practice may itself offer you insights in what you can handle.

Regular deep breathing can help you hone your focus. Eventually, you might be in a position to meditate in occupied and loud situations.

Practice mindfulness. One important way of improving your meditation practice is to activate in mindfulness during your day. Rather than allowing your anxieties to distract you from the world around you, concentrate on the here and today. Focus on things that you do in today's and individuals you are with. Having the ability to stay present can help you strengthen your concentrate by restricting negative considering and panic.

Training mindfulness also may help improve your feeling and lessen stress. Look after your body. Keeping your physical health can be an important step towards developing your practice. For a while, you should stretch out prior to meditating to avoid cramping or pain throughout your practice. In the long run, make an effort to eat healthy and live a dynamic life. This will make sure that you are physically able to develop and grow in your meditation practice. Being disciplined about your daily diet and exercise may offer you understood discoveries about yourself. Be patient. It's important to identify that you'll not immediately reach a spot of self-awareness and breakthrough. It requires lots of time and practice. In fact, deep breathing alone won't help you better understand yourself. Meditation, in mixture with daily mindfulness methods, can help you reach your goal of self-discovery.

Consider guided meditation. If you're having a hard time concentrating on your own, a led deep breathing can help you begin. Within this practice, a skilled specialist verbally manuals you through the meditation process. This assists you focus on your concentrate by allowing your brain to relax and follow another person as they business lead you through the practice. You can find sound and video clips of guided practices online. There's also led deep breathing songs on Spotify.

Promoting Self-Discovery through Every day Practices

Give consideration. Be intentional about focusing on whatever you do. If you're eating and taking in, do no watch Television or take a look at your mobile phone. Instead, concentrate on the feelings of the meals. Also, completely take part in discussions with others. This can help you be considered a more empathic and conscientious participant when you connect to others. By concentrating on the items you do, you shall gain insights about yourself. Such as, can you focus on a conversation or are you easily unfocused?

Do normal things in various ways. If you perform a task every day in a certain way, try changing it a bit. This might offer you a new way of taking a look at your activities and exactly how you undertake the world.

In the event that you regularly walk to work along a certain path, try going another real way.

In the event that you typically perform an activity with your right hands, check it out with your remaining.

Practice your deep breathing. Throughout your day, make an effort to focus on your respiration just like you were meditating. This can help you relax and become better in a position to take in today's. You are able to practice this when you are seated at your table, standing in collection at the supermarket, or on your bus trip home.

Even twenty mere seconds of gradual and rhythmic deep breathing can help you gain some mental space and just a little perspective.

Engage your senses. Absorb your body as well as your sense's reactions to stimuli. Focus about how things flavor, smell, audio, feel and appearance. Investigate any thoughts or feelings that might arise from certain sensations. This may help you develop some personal insights.

For instance, eat one of your preferred foods and focus on the feelings that you are feeling. These sensations might help clarify why you like this food and dislike others, which can result in revelations about who you are.

Be curious. Investigate the global world around you. Explore new encounters and push yourself to try different things. Examine your reactions to these new experiences and situations. Try to realize why you love certain things over others and what that says about you. An elevated fascination with the world around will help unlock insights about who you are.

This might also help you feel a far more empathic and thoughtful person.

Chapter 28: SECTION SEVEN

POST-TRAUMATIC STRESS DISORDER (PTSD);

MEANING AND CAUSES

It's not uncommon for people who have experienced traumatic events to have flashbacks, nightmares, or intrusive memories when something terrible happens like the 9/11 terrorist attacks and those in cities around the world (Orlando and Paris, for instance) or the bombings at the 2013 Boston Marathon, or active combat.

Posttraumatic stress disorder, or PTSD, is a serious potentially devastating condition that can occur in people who have experienced or witnessed a traumatic event such as natural disaster, serious accident, terrorist incident, unexpected death of a loved one, war, rape, or other life-threatening events, a physical brain injury, specifically of damaged tissue.

Most people who witness such events recover from them, but people with PTSD continue to be severely depressed and anxious for months or even years following the event.

Anyone can develop PTSD at any age. Women are twice as likely to develop posttraumatic stress disorder as men, and children can also develop it. PTSD often arises with depression, substance abuse, or other anxiety disorders.

It is natural to feel afraid during and after a traumatic condition. Fear activates many split-second changes in the

body to help defend against danger or to avoid it. This "fight-or-flight" response is a typical reaction meant to protect a person from harm.

It is important to remember that not everyone who lives through a dangerous event develops PTSD. In fact, most people will not develop the disorder. Nearly everyone will experience a range of reactions after trauma, yet most people recover from initial symptoms naturally. Persons who continue to experience problems may be diagnosed with PTSD. People who have PTSD may feel stressed or frightened even when they are not in danger.

SIGNS AND SYMPTOMS OF POST-TRAUMATIC STRESS DISORDER (PTSD);

Symptoms usually begin early, within 3 months of the traumatic incident, but sometimes they begin years later. Symptoms must last more than a month and be severe enough to interfere with relationships or work to be considered PTSD. The course of the illness differs. Some people recover within 6 months, while some others have symptoms that last much longer. In some people, the condition becomes chronic.

Anyone can develop PTSD at any age. This includes war veterans, children, and individuals who have been through a physical or sexual assault, abuse, accident, disaster, or many other serious events.

It is important to remember that not everyone who lives through a dangerous event develops PTSD. In fact, most people will not develop the disorder.

To be diagnosed with PTSD, an adult must have all of the following symptoms for at least 1 month:

- No less than two arousal and reactivity symptoms

- No less than two cognition and mood symptoms

- No less than one re-experiencing symptom

- No less than one avoidance symptom

Arousal and reactivity symptoms include:

Being easily startled

Feeling tense or "on edge"

Having difficulty sleeping

Having angry outbursts

Cognition and mood symptoms include:

Trouble remembering key features of the traumatic event

Negative thoughts about oneself or the world

Distorted feelings like guilt or blame

Loss of interest in enjoyable activities

Re-experiencing symptoms include:

Flashbacks

Bad dreams

Frightening thoughts

Avoidance symptoms include:

Staying away from places, events, or objects that are reminders of the traumatic experience

Avoiding thoughts or feelings related to the traumatic event.

It is natural to have some of these symptoms after a dangerous incident. Sometimes people have very serious symptoms that go away after a few weeks. This is called acute stress disorder, or ASD.

When the symptoms last more than one month, seriously affect one's ability to function, and are not due to substance use, medical illness, or anything except the event itself, they might be PTSD. Some people with PTSD do not show any symptoms for weeks or months. PTSD often go with depression, substance abuse, or one or more of the other anxiety disorders.

Children and teens can have extreme reactions to trauma, but their symptoms may not be the same as adults. In very young children (less than six years of age), these symptoms can include:

Forgetting how to or being unable to talk

Acting out the scary event during playtime

Being unusually clingy with a parent or other adult

Wetting the bed after having learned to use the toilet

Older children and teens are more likely to display symptoms similar to those seen in adults. They may also develop troublesome, disrespectful, or destructive conducts. Older children and teens may feel guilt-ridden for not preventing injury or deaths. They may also have thoughts of retaliation.

MANAGEMENT OF POST-TRAUMATIC STRESS DISORDER (PTSD);

The chief treatments for people with PTSD are medications, psychotherapy ("talk" therapy), or both.

Identify and seek out comforting conditions, people and places.

discuss with your doctor about treatment options

Participate in mild physical activity or exercise to help reduce stress

Set realistic goals for yourself

Expect your symptoms to improve gradually, not instantly.

Break up large tasks into smaller pieces, set some priorities, and do what you can as you can.

Try to spend time with other people, and Tell trusted friends or relatives about things that may trigger symptoms.

Chapter 29: How to sleep well again

First and foremost, do take note to avoid using sleeping pills or alcohol to aid you in sleeping. Those will often lead to dependence, and there is a high potential of abuse. Only use sleeping pills when prescribed by a doctor!

Everybody's a little different, so understand that you should be patient and try out all the different techniques before being frustrated once more. With that being said, here are some tips you can follow to curb the long nights.

✽ ✽ ✽

Healthy sleeping habits

This is pretty obvious of course but it's a huge factor in most people's sleep.

A good night's sleep can have a big impact on your feelings and performance the next day. Getting your beauty sleep regularly, makes you feel less tired, tense or irritated at the smallest things.

Sleep not only helps to repair our physical body, but it also helps to improve our processing of information. On the other hand, poor sleep **leads to a weaker immune system and several mental problems such as anxiety and depression**. It is common that a mental illness is linked to several others, and this emphasizes the importance of positive mental health.

In order to overcome insomnia, we will have to get rid of our bad sleeping habits. Bad habits like using the phone on the bed, or watching late night shows can affect the quality of your sleep.

Good sleep practices include being in a dark and comfortable environment. New sheets, an air freshener, etc will help with being at ease. An advice for all is to adjust the lighting, temperature and noise level in your bedroom.

The perfect bedroom atmosphere suggested would be to have low levels of lighting and noise, and warm temperature. However, different people have different preferences for their perfect bedroom atmosphere. Some may fall asleep faster with white noises playing in the background, or to sleep in an air-conditioned room.

Only use the bed for sleeping, as it is a form of stimulus control. You can condition the body to know when to sleep, but you need discipline! If you fail to sleep within 20 minutes, stop and try to tire yourself out doing other meditative activities, like writing a diary or meditating.

All these require a certain level of commitment, but it's worth doing to get your beauty sleep!

There has been an increase in demand for weighted blankets recently, and I have also jumped on the bandwagon to purchase one. Although not completely backed by strong scientific claims, weighted blankets offer a very compelling choice for people who have trouble sleeping. Being hugged all night sounds awesome and from a logical and anecdotal standpoint, it really makes sense. It's been documented by a few individuals that using weighted blankets helped them fall asleep faster, for longer hours and felt more refreshed to start the day. Sounds just like the right thing we ALL need, regardless if we have insomnia or not!

For those suffering from insomnia for quite a while, perhaps changing your bedroom atmosphere can't be of much help. A solution for you may be to explore Cognitive Behavioral Therapy (CBT) through a professional's recommendation.

✷ ✷ ✷

Exercise

While a good jog in the day would release chemicals that'll allow you to have a more restful sleep, there's more to it! Our bodies have a circadian rhythm, think of it like a bio-clock. It is very sensitive to light, so a morning jog will allow your body to fully wake up and sync to the rotation of the sun.

This makes it easier to sleep at designated timings when you have a scheduled lifestyle. A worked out body will naturally crave sleep. Quick, hit the gym!

✱ ✱ ✱

Avoid drugs or caffeine

Drugs have been known to alter the sleep and resting hours of individuals significantly. More common forms of chemical usage includes smoking and drinking coffee. Avoiding those activities in the evening helps a lot with sleeping regularly! Remember, it's always good advice to quit smoking!

Caffeine has been named the most popular drug in the world. All over the world, people consume caffeine on a daily basis in coffee, tea, cocoa, chocolate, some soft drinks, and some drugs. But I would recommend those who are suffering from insomnia to stop getting your caffeine fix.

Because caffeine is a stimulant, most people would use it to wake up for early mornings or to remain alert during the rest of the day. The experience by people with insomnia would be to consume more caffeine to stay awake for the rest of the day, but it also causes a vicious cycle of sleeplessness.

Caffeine disrupts your sleep. This makes you rely more heavily on caffeine, which makes it that much harder to sleep the next night. Breaking this cycle of dependency on caffeine can help your sleep and make you feel less fatigued and more focused during the day.

As a first step to stopping your caffeine addiction, check the timings that you consume a cup of coffee. I would recommend to stop all caffeinated drinks at 2.pm. If you usually consume coffee in the afternoon, switch to decaf. If you're craving to have a post-dinner cup of coffee with your friend, try swapping that with a cup of tea. Timing is really important because caffeine has a long lasting impact after consumption, between 6-8 hours. This means that it probably takes eight hours for all that caffeine to be metabolized by your body. Cutting your coffee consumption at 2pm ensures that you'll be able to start falling asleep by 1030pm!

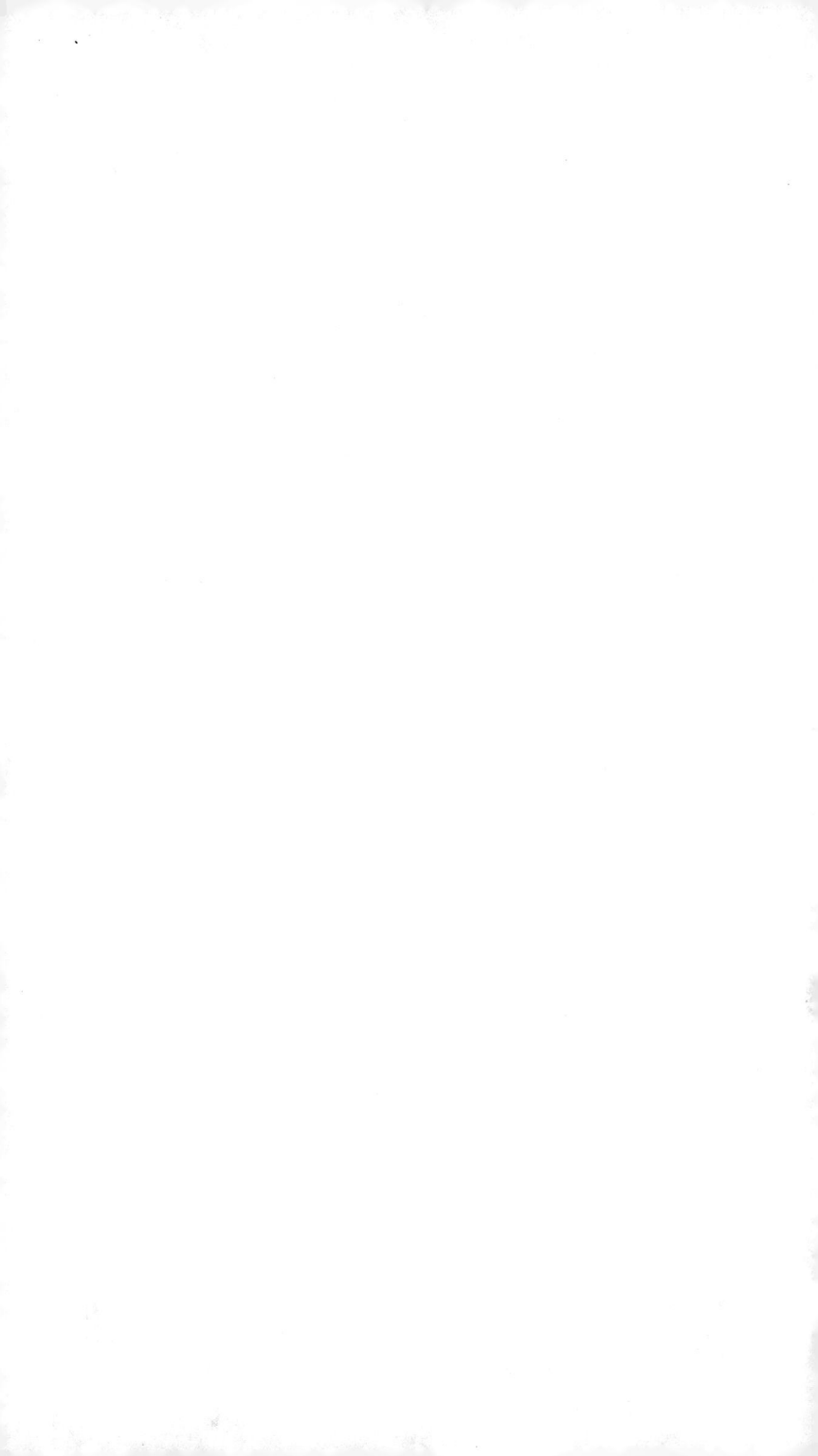

CPSIA information can be obtained
at www.ICGtesting.com
Printed in the USA
BVHW032255261022
650444BV00010B/85

9 781989 920657